Neuropsychology for Occupational Therapists

Cognition in Occupational Performance

Third Edition

June Grieve
BSc, MSc

Linda Gnanasekaran
MSc, BSc (Hons), DipCOT FHEA

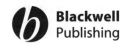

Blackwell
Publishing

Blackwell Publishing editorial offices:
Blackwell Publishing Ltd, 9600
Garsington Road, Oxford OX4 2DQ, UK
Tel: +44 (0)1865 776868
Blackwell Publishing Inc., 350 Main Street, Malden, MA 02148-5020, USA
Tel: +1 781 388 8250
Blackwell Publishing Asia Pty Ltd, 550 Swanston Street, Carlton, Victoria 3053, Australia
Tel: +61 (0)3 8359 1011

First published 2008 by Blackwell Publishing Ltd

ISBN-13: 978-1-4051-3699-0

Library of Congress Cataloging-in-Publication Data

Grieve, June I.
    Neuropsychology for occupational therapists : cognition in
occupational performance / June Grieve, Linda Gnanasekaran. – 3rd ed.
        p. ; cm.
    Includes bibliographical references and index.
    ISBN-13: 978-1-4051-3699-0 (pbk. : alk. paper)
    1. Clinical neuropsychology.   2. Cognition disorders–Patients–
Rehabilitation.   3. Occupational therapy.   I. Gnanasekaran, Linda.   II. Title.
    [DNLM: 1. Neuropsychology.   2. Cognition–physiology.   3. Cognition
Disorders–diagnosis.   4. Memory Disorders–diagnosis.   5. Neurologic
Examination.   6. Occupational Therapy.   7. Perception–physiology. WL
103.5 G848n 2007]
    RC386.6.N48G75 2007
    616.8′0475–dc22
                                                                        2007037064

A catalogue record for this title is available from the British Library

Set in 9.5 on 12.5 pt Palatino by SNP Best-set Typesetter Ltd., Hong Kong

Printed and bound in Singapore by Fabulous Printers Pte Ltd

The publisher's policy is to use permanent paper from mills that operate a sustainable forestry policy, and which has been manufactured from pulp processed using acid-free and elementary chlorine-free practices. Furthermore, the publisher ensures that the text paper and cover board used have met acceptable environmental accreditation standards.

For further information on Blackwell Publishing, visit our website:
www.blackwellpublishing.com

Contents

Preface

This book was written primarily for undergraduate students of occupational therapy. Experienced clinicians will find a useful review of frameworks used within the profession to structure assessment and intervention, together with an update of knowledge in neuropsychology. Members of the multidisciplinary team will gain an insight into the unique role of the occupational therapist in cognitive rehabilitation. The first edition of *Neuropsychology for Occupational Therapists* was written at the time when cognitive rehabilitation was becoming one of the major areas of occupational therapy practice. The aim was to create an understanding of the part played by cognition, and the effects of its impairment, in daily living.

Relevant assessments of perception and cognition were presented and developed further in the second edition to reflect an increase in the number of standardised assessments available. Now, in this third edition, Linda Gnanasekaran has related the study of cognitive functions and impairment to current occupational therapy practice. Part 1 introduces cognition within the context of occupational performance, emphasising its pivotal role. An occupational focus for cognitive rehabilitation is proposed, based upon two theoretical frameworks: one an internationally recognised model of health; the other specific to occupational therapy. The value of these frameworks is explored in relation to the occupational therapy process, exemplifying how theoretical constructs, core skills and knowledge are combined to achieve a rigorous approach to rehabilitation. Not only the student or novice practitioner, but also experienced clinicians, are given a succinct review of the occupational therapy process. Part 1 establishes the therapeutic context for the knowledge presented in Part 2.

Part 2 outlines the theoretical background for each of the components of the cognitive system and describes the disorders associated with their impairment. The presentation of cognitive function in separate chapters facilitates the discussion of relevant research in neuropsychology. It must, however, be remembered that occupational therapists are often confronted with people who present with multiple impairments.

Activities in earlier editions, which encourage the reader to focus on their own cognitive abilities, have been retained and extended. The introduction of case studies and summaries of functional consequences of disorders reinforces the effects of impairment on function. Part 2 carries over the general guidelines given in Part 1 to suggestions for assessment and intervention related to specific areas of cognition. Our task of integrating basic knowledge with occupational therapy has proved daunting and exciting. If this text is found useful as a resource for neuropsychology, and for guidance to practice, then we have achieved our aims.

June Grieve and Linda Gnanasekaran

Acknowledgements

We would like to express our thanks to Stephanie Tempest who gave us help and advice in many ways, based on her clinical and teaching experience. In particular, we thank Stephanie for writing Chapter 9 on Purposeful Movement and Apraxia, and for her contributions to the suggestions for assessment and intervention.

We also wish to thank Jo Creighton, who continued her artistic endeavours which began in the first two editions of the book. Jo devised and produced all the original drawings in Part 1 and updated several in Part 2.

Extracts from the Rivermead Perceptual Assessment Battery are included by permission of the publishers, NFER-NELSON, The Chiswick Centre, 414 Chiswick High Road, London W4 5TF. The extract from the Chessington Occupational Therapy Assessment Battery is included with permission of Nottingham Rehab Supplies, Victoria Business Park, Pintail Close, Netherfield, Nottingham NG4 2PE. The extract from the Behavioural Inattention Test is included with permission of Harcourt Assessment, Halley Court, Jordan Hill, Oxford OX2 8EJ.

Part 1 Cognition and the Occupational Therapy Process

Part 1 delineates and describes the practice of occupational therapy in relation to the needs of people with cognitive impairments. It consists of three chapters.

Chapter 1 establishes that cognition is a fundamental component of all purposeful activity and presents an occupational rationale for addressing cognitive problems. The reader is introduced to two theoretical frameworks. One describes the domain of occupational therapy and its components and processes. The other is an international framework that defines and articulates components of health and well-being. Together they are used to conceptualise and structure the role and functions of occupational therapy in cognitive rehabilitation.

Chapter 2 proceeds to discuss the purpose and practice of assessment in cognitive rehabilitation. Frameworks are reviewed in terms of their value for assessment, and good assessment practices and procedures are described. Key factors are considered which contribute to sound clinical reasoning and decision making, in order to achieve appropriate assessment.

Chapter 3 presents a comprehensive overview of the intervention process and considers issues of evaluating the outcomes of intervention. Rehabilitation interventions are considered in terms of context and suitability of approaches. A range of common methods and techniques are briefly described, along with considerations of how to grade interventions.

Throughout Part 1, the intention is to present general guidelines, considerations and recommendations for practice. Neither a prescriptive set of assessment and intervention solutions to specific cognitive problems, nor ready-made 'recipes' for practice will be presented. Every therapist must utilise their own knowledge, reasoning and professional skills to provide the best possible occupational therapy for each of their clients. Part 1 aims to provide support to that process.

The general guidelines for assessment and intervention given in Chapters 2 and 3 should be considered in conjunction with the more detailed suggestions given at the end of Chapters 5–10.

1 Occupation and Cognitive Rehabilitation

The scope of cognitive rehabilitation

Occupation is described as being 'purposeful or meaningful activities in which humans engage as part of their normal daily lives . . . all aspects of living that contribute to health and fulfilment for an individual' (McColl *et al.*, 2003, p. 1). It has been more broadly defined as 'everything people do to occupy themselves including looking after themselves and contributing to the social and economic fabric of their communities' (Law *et al.*, 1997, p. 32).

That any health problem can have implications for all aspects of life, and not just the physical and mental state of the individual, is becoming an accepted view. It is endorsed and embodied within the World Health Organisation's definition of health as 'a state of complete physical, mental and social well-being and not merely the absence of disease or infirmity' (World Health Organisation, 1946). By accepting the definitions of occupation given above, it can be appreciated that the occupational components of an individual's life become central to health and well-being.

For individuals with neurological damage, cognitive deficits are often the source of functional problems but they are unseen or difficult to manage. Poor task performance, in the absence of motor deficits, may originate in poor object recognition or sequencing (see Figure 1.1). The person who cannot recognise his or her family may be mistakenly labelled with memory loss. The person who does not respond to questions may have an attention problem which is often confused with deafness. Also, there are several possible reasons which account for a person who lives alone being unable to organise a daily routine.

Disorders of brain structure or function, inherited or acquired, may give rise to difficulties in the ways that people think, feel and/or act. These difficulties can result in loss of, or difficulties in acquiring or maintaining, abilities and skills. This results in changes in the social, economic and home circumstances of

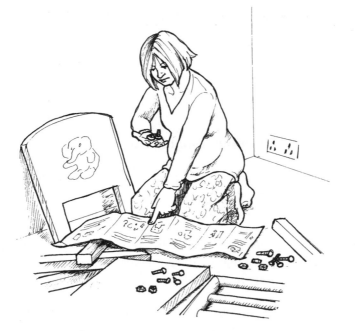

Fig. 1.1 Cognitive deficits result in problems with task performance.

the individual and his family. Within the context of occupation, cognitive deficits are likely to impact on some, if not all aspects of life, and occupational therapy forms a significant component of rehabilitation.

Occupational therapists engage with people as patients, clients, students, workers and family members, in a range of environments such as hospitals, day centres, schools, the workplace and the home. Hence, occupational assessment becomes paramount to investigate the full impact of cognitive deficits upon the life of the affected individual, and also upon the people he/she relates and interacts with.

The scope of cognitive rehabilitation arguably embraces virtually all aspects of life. Assessment is only one part of a process that seeks to enable an individual to function optimally within his or her usual environment(s), to maintain health and well-being, and engage in valued occupations (Crepeau *et al.*, 2003). The causes (for example traumatic brain injury, cerebrovascular disease, infection) and nature of cognitive deficits may require intermittent or long-term engagement with rehabilitation and/or support services, at any point in life.

Cognition, occupation and the International Classification of Functioning, Disability and Health

Effective therapeutic intervention requires a means of gathering and organising information (a *framework*). This needs to address not only neurological functioning, but also the individual's capacity for and ability to engage in necessary and valued occupations. It requires the means to address the interrelationship of the person and his/her occupations with the environments and contexts in which they occur.

Occupational therapists have become accustomed to working within frameworks derived from theoretical models of practice and theories of human occupation. In parallel, over the last few decades, the World Health Organisation (WHO) has been working towards a framework for the definition and classification of all aspects of health and related factors.

The International Classification of Functioning, Disability and Health (ICF) (WHO, 2001) is a multi-purpose system of classification developed through international collaboration, that codifies health and health related aspects of human life. Its chief aim is to provide a common language of concepts, definitions and terms for examining health and the individual's ability to function. It is designed to do so in a way that provides for:

- Clear communication between professionals, agencies, the public and service users
- Comparison of data from disparate sources (different countries, different health care disciplines)
- Systematic coding for health information systems

In doing so, the ICF also provides a framework for systematic examination of the relationship between disorders of health, the ability to undertake occupations and the interaction of the individual with the environment.

The ICF is introduced here as a means to facilitate and enhance the assessment, rehabilitation and support of people with cognitive deficits. It is a *biopsychosocial* framework that considers health in relation to activities, participation, environmental and other factors. It therefore allows a holistic and comprehensive approach to identifying, measuring and treating health-related difficulties for any individual.

The ICF is structured in two parts. Part 1 classifies and defines *body structures* and *functions*, and human *activities* and *participation* (in life situations). Part 2 classifies and defines *contexts* of human function – *environmental* (external influences) and *personal* (or internal influences). Figure 1.2 gives an overview of the major components of the ICF.

The comprehensive and precise qualities of the ICF provide the potential for it to be used as a basis for the development of accurate evaluation tools that can measure the interactions of an individual's disability with all aspects of his/her life. Within each component of the ICF, all terms are clearly defined and broken down further. All elements are coded, so that, for example, within the component of 'Body functions' we find 'Mental functions: Global mental functions', within which b110 is the code for 'Consciousness functions' defined as 'General mental functions of the state of awareness and alertness, including the clarity and continuity of the wakeful state' (WHO, 2001, p. 48).

From a rehabilitation perspective, the ICF categorises and codifies all components of a person's life that could be affected by health status, or could in turn have an effect upon health. In the

Part One: Functioning and disability		
• Components	Body Functions: These encompass all physiological functions of body systems (including psychological functions)	
	Body structures: These encompass all anatomical parts of the body such as organs, limbs and their components	
	Impairment: This term refers to any problems in body function or structure such as significant deviation or loss	
	Activity: is the execution of a task or action by an individual	
	Participation: is involvement in a life situation	
	Activity limitations: Difficulties in executing activities	
	Participation restrictions: difficulties with involvement in life situations	
Part Two: Contextual factors		
• Components	Environmental factors: external influences on functioning and disability (physical, interpersonal, societal etc)	
	Personal factors: internal influences on functioning and disability not related to health (gender, age, life experiences etc).These are not classified but may contribute to and impact upon functioning and disability	

Fig. 1.2 The International Classification of Functioning, Disability and Health (WHO, 2001): components and definitions.

case of persons with impairments of cognitive functions, it facilitates the assessment of, and planning interventions for, consequent activity limitations and participation restrictions.

Table 1.1 presents an example of how the framework could be used to track the relationship between impairments of body structure and function, through to activities and participation and relevant contextual factors, for an individual with an acquired brain injury.

Measurement of such interactions between biological, environmental and personal factors, to result in a particular level of functioning, has been considered lacking in the field of neuropsychology (Bilbao *et al.*, 2003). Many of the studies of cognitive function in neuropsychology are laboratory based and may not take into account the person's gender, occupation or lifestyle. However, over recent years there has been a move to increase ecological validity in studies in psychology. Investigations of memory, topographical orientation and executive functions, in particular, have measured the responses of both normal and brain damaged people during everyday living (Shallice & Burgess, 1991). Also, in single case studies in cognitive neuropsychology, a full case history of the person is given. It is hoped that a greater awareness and understanding of cognitive function, and the use of systematic frameworks like the ICF, will enhance measurement and understanding of the impact of cognitive deficits upon function.

The ICF in relation to occupational therapy

Within its framework, the ICF includes all those human activities, tasks and roles that conventionally fall within the professional domain of concern of occupational therapists. The College of Occupational Therapists (UK) considers that the ICF usefully 'shifts the concept of health and disability from cause to impact by considering the issues and problems for individuals within their own context rather than by medical diagnosis' (COT, 2005, p. 3) (see Figure 1.3). In support of this assertion, it can be seen that the classifications used by the ICF usefully parallel current occupational therapy concepts and definitions of humans as occupational beings. Frameworks of practice utilised by occupational therapists bear significant similarities to large sections of the ICF, making it possible to translate profession-specific findings and information into *and* draw such information out of this multi-agency, multidisciplinary and internationally recognised format. This is illustrated

Table 1.1   An example of the categories of the ICF used to organise and track the possible consequences, difficulties and contextual issues for an individual with an acquired brain injury.

Body functions *for example	Body structures *for example
Global mental functions:	*Structures of the nervous system:*
Orientation	Structure of brain
Intellect	Frontal lobe
Specific mental functions:	Parietal lobe
Attention	Temporal lobe
Memory	Occipital lobe
Thought	
Higher-level cognitive functions	

Impairments of brain structures and functions will take the form of deficits or changes, for example *loss* of cortical tissue, *in*attention, *dis*orientation, etc. In turn, impairments may affect activities and participation (capacity for and/or performance of) giving rise to **activity limitations** and **participation restrictions . . .**

Activities and participation *for example	
Learning and applying knowledge:	*General tasks and demands:*
Acquiring complex skills	Undertaking a complex task
Thinking	Undertaking multiple tasks
Reading and writing	
Solving problems	
Making decisions	
Community, social and civic life:	*Work and employment:*
Engaging in hobbies	Maintaining a job
Socialising	

. . . such limitations and restrictions, their impact and importance, would be affected by other factors. Similarly, other factors could be manipulated to mitigate the effect of impairments upon activities and participation.

Environmental factors *for example	
Products and technology:	*Support and relationships:*
For communication	Immediate family
For employment	Friends
	People in positions of authority

* Every component and sub-component of the ICF has a detailed definition and a code number. These enable precision and clarity of understanding, recording and communicating of information. This table only gives selected examples of some categories of the ICF that would be relevant in this case.

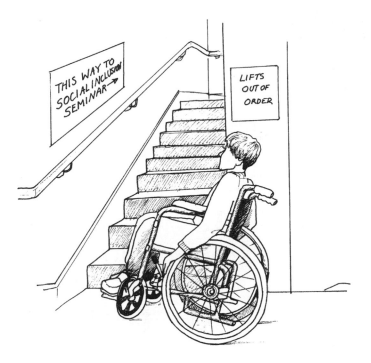

Fig. 1.3 Medical diagnosis is not the only barrier to participation.

in Table 1.2, where comparisons are drawn between the ICF and one of the commonly used occupational therapy frameworks, the Occupational Therapy Practice Framework (OTPF) produced by the American Occupational Therapy Association (AOT, 2002). The ICF and the OTPF will be used as the frameworks that inform our discussions about the role and functions of occupational therapy in cognitive rehabilitation.

Because of its multi-purpose, multi-professional nature, the ICF cannot incorporate all possible variations upon categorisation of the human state, since each health care profession will require focus and specificity upon different aspects, and will need its own language and concepts for this. Table 1.2 illustrates how the OTPF specifies the need for occupational therapists to analyse activities in terms of their properties and demands upon the individual, as well as the individual's ability to perform the activity. Hence, *performance skills*, *performance patterns* and *activity demands* are components of and demands upon human functioning that do not map neatly onto the ICF framework. However, they reflect the enhanced detail and performance-related information needed by occupational therapists in the analysis of an individual's functional needs and performance difficulties.

Table 1.2 Illustration of the relationship between the ICF and a current practice framework used in occupational therapy (Occupational Therapy Practice Framework, AOTA, 2002).

ICF	Body functions and body structures	Activities and participation	Environmental factors	Personal factors
Categories correspond to:				
Occupational Therapy Practice Framework	Client factors Body functions and body structures	Areas of occupation Activities of daily living Instrumental ADL Education Work, play, leisure Social participation	Performance contexts Physical Social Temporal Virtual	Spiritual Personal
Additional components identified in the AOTA Practice Framework, not found in the ICF	{············· Performance skills ·················} Motor skills Process skills / Communication/interaction skills	{·········· Performance patterns ·········} Habits Routines Roles		
	{················ Activity Demands ················} Required actions / Objects and their properties / Space demands Sequence and timing / Social demands Required body structures and function			

Applying theoretical frameworks

Most students and practitioners of occupational therapy use a range of theoretical models and frameworks to delineate, organise and understand the occupational needs and problems of the individuals and groups of people that they work with. In the preceding sections of this chapter, the ICF was introduced and compared to the OTPF. These two frameworks help us to organise large and sometimes quite disparate amounts of information in a systematic way, and to identify the relationships between them. What these frameworks *do not* do is provide theories or explanations about *why* a particular phenomenon or relationship exists; nor do they promote or guide the therapist as to tools, methods or techniques they might use to address an individual's occupational needs and problems. These latter functions are served by theories of cognition, rehabilitation and the tenets of the occupational therapy profession. These are referred to further in Chapter 3.

The use and value of the ICF and OTPF can be illustrated by the use of a case example. First, the applicability of the ICF will be considered.

Case study

Mr B is a 35-year-old man who sustained a traumatic brain injury when he was knocked off his bicycle by a car. He sustained some soft tissue injuries (bruising and cuts) but these resolved quite quickly. He worked serving customers in a fast food restaurant, and lived with his parents. Mr B was discharged home after two weeks in hospital, and referred to the community occupational therapy team. At initial interview Mr B identified some difficulties with his memory. His parents had observed changes to his behaviour – a lack of initiative in self-care and domestic tasks, and a tendency to be forgetful and easily distracted from the task in hand – which Mr B did not acknowledge. Further specific assessments identified some difficulties with recall and recognition, problem solving, abstract thinking and calculation. Other aspects of cognition, for example short-term memory, sequencing and simple maths skills were within normal limits.

Using the ICF framework, these cognitive impairments and their implications for occupational performance can be organised and identified in relationship to each other and to the contextual factors of Mr B's life (see Figure 1.4.).

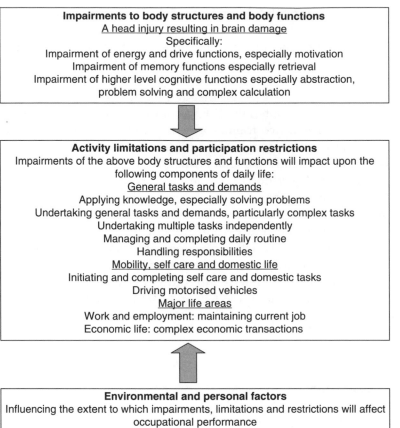

Impairments to body structures and body functions
A head injury resulting in brain damage
Specifically:
Impairment of energy and drive functions, especially motivation
Impairment of memory functions especially retrieval
Impairment of higher level cognitive functions especially abstraction,
problem solving and complex calculation

Activity limitations and participation restrictions
Impairments of the above body structures and functions will impact upon the
following components of daily life:
General tasks and demands
Applying knowledge, especially solving problems
Undertaking general tasks and demands, particularly complex tasks
Undertaking multiple tasks independently
Managing and completing daily routine
Handling responsibilities
Mobility, self care and domestic life
Initiating and completing self care and domestic tasks
Driving motorised vehicles
Major life areas
Work and employment: maintaining current job
Economic life: complex economic transactions

Environmental and personal factors
Influencing the extent to which impairments, limitations and restrictions will affect
occupational performance

Environmental
Immediate family support
Home situation – living with others
Availability of transport
Community facilities
Employment opportunities

Personal
Emotional response to his
situation
Personal values and life goals
Awareness of own capacity
and performance
Interpersonal skills

Fig. 1.4 Illustration of the use of the ICF to delineate activity limitations and participation restrictions arising from a head injury.

Why are frameworks useful?

This case example shows the use of the ICF framework and descriptors to identify in a systematic way how a change in health status impacts upon Mr B's occupational performance. From this point the unique skills and knowledge of occupational therapy are essential to explore, understand and diagnose the interaction of these elements as well as their individual contributions to his difficulties. In addition to the basic framework of components and definitions, the ICF identifies two components of any individual's activity and participation that together determine his/her ability; these are termed *capacity* and *performance.*

'Capacity' is a qualifier which refers to a person's *capability*, that is their highest or best level of performance in a standardised environment (for example in a laboratory or rehabilitation kitchen). 'Performance' refers to a person's *actual* performance within the contexts of their normal environment (for example in their local shop or their own kitchen). In Mr B's case, he may be able to produce a cooked meal within the familiar environs of his own kitchen due to being prompted by visual and contextual cues that are present, but may be unable to do so in an unfamiliar rehabilitation kitchen. This highlights the importance of assessing both components of an individual's abilities, as limited capacity for a particular activity would not necessarily predict limited performance. Conversely, successful performance of an activity could not be assumed to indicate normal capacity.

Applying this issue to clinical practice, a neuropsychological test of object recognition might identify a limitation in this cognitive process. This would need further exploration in the person's usual environment and contexts to determine the extent and impact of the deficit.

Why an occupational therapy framework is important for effective rehabilitation

The ICF identifies capacity and performance as dimensions of carrying out activities and participation. It also acknowledges the influence that contexts may have upon the individual's situation (for example physical environment or economic status) and identifies that these can either act as *facilitators* or *barriers* to a person's ability to function (WHO, 2001). But beyond the definitions of capacity and performance, the ICF does not offer any further framework for the analysis of human abilities. It does suggest measurement scales for rating levels of impairment, activity limitation and participation restriction, but these are generic and do not allow for describing the nature of a problem in any given area. It allows description of a difficulty but not diagnosis of its precise nature or cause.

Occupational therapists therefore need an *occupational* framework to further identify and diagnose the precise nature of an individual's occupational difficulties – and strengths – in order to plan effective treatment or other interventions. The OTPF (see Table 1.2 above) provides a structure by which:

- The demands an activity makes upon an individual can be further defined
- The environmental aspects can be fully analysed
- The performance skills and patterns a person needs to carry them out can be analysed

Without such knowledge, it would be difficult to analyse fully the impact of any given impairment (of body structure or function) upon an individual's occupational performance. To illustrate this, let us consider the example of driving a car. Most adults have a general appreciation of what driving a car entails and the skills it requires, whether or not they know how to drive. Most of us, if asked, would identify that driving requires the ability to:

- Coordinate upper and lower limbs
- See clearly
- Know and apply the rules and laws of the road
- Operate the controls of a car

However, what are less obvious are the *demands* the activity makes upon the individual in terms of their performance skills, and how contexts can influence these. Such performance skills would include the ability to:

- Maintain energy and an effective pace of performance
- Sustain attention and selectively attend to important visual, auditory and tactile information
- Utilise knowledge (using short-term, procedural and topographical memory) to achieve a desired goal (reach destination safely)
- Organise self and the immediate environment for effective operation of the car
- Initiate, sequence and terminate the tasks involved in driving appropriately
- Maintain position and produce coordinated sequences of movements, working bilaterally and unilaterally to operate controls
- Notice, respond and adjust to changing conditions and unexpected events

The extent to which these performance skills are needed or used at any time in a period of driving would change according to the

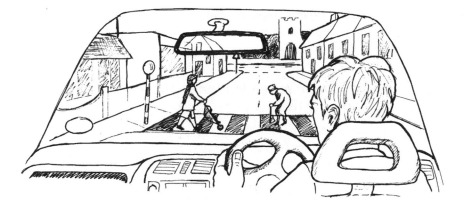

Fig. 1.5   Driving a car makes multiple demands upon the individual.

road conditions, local geography and the actions of other road users (see Figure 1.5).

The OTPF identifies performance *skills*, performance *patterns*, and activity *demands* as being dimensions, emphasising that it is not only the individual's personal attributes (body structures and functions) that determine ability, but the environment and characteristics of the activity or role itself that are important to its execution. This highlights three things:

1. Occupational therapy emphasises performance rather than capacity; that is the person's ability to 'do' or function in his or her normal environments and contexts.
2. Occupational therapists recognise that the nature, content and context of an activity will also influence how it is performed, and therefore affect the demands it makes of an individual.
3. When working to resolve a person's occupational difficulties, it is not just the individual's own health and abilities that need to be addressed but also the contextual aspects of his or her performance, because these may be acting as *facilitators* or *barriers* to performance.

Hence, it can be seen that combining the two frameworks provides a systematic mechanism by which the occupational therapist can:

• Analyse the characteristics and demands of any given task, activity or occupation

- Determine the individual's impairments, activity limitations and participation restrictions that need further investigation and assessment

Why knowledge of cognition is needed for analysing occupations, tasks and activities

The individual mental processes that constitute cognition involve complex neural mechanisms in themselves (perception or memory, for example), but always operate within a larger complex of integrated and interrelating functions. Perception requires memory, because without memory we would not learn what objects are, and therefore we would not be able to recognise them. Conversely, establishing memories requires perception, because without perceptual processing we could not attach meaning to an experience.

Let us return to the example of driving a car, and think about the activity of driving down a busy street. The driver will need a mental map of the route he is taking. This requires memory, and the ability to constantly take in the scene around him and compare it to his 'mental map', in order to know how far he has got. In other words he must be able to perceive incoming visual information, integrate it with stored knowledge, and use this to plan his next actions.

In addition, he must at all times maintain attention to the activity of driving the car, using the controls and checking his speed and position on the road. He must monitor events around him; pedestrians, other vehicles, traffic lights and signs. He may also simultaneously be conversing with a passenger or listening to a radio.

To achieve all this, our driver must be capable of:

- Attention – sustained, selective and shifting
- Perception – visuo-spatial, auditory, tactile
- Use of short-term, procedural and topographical memory
- Motor planning and execution of skilled movements
- Executive functions: problem solving and rapid decision making

This analysis of driving demonstrates the fundamental importance of cognitive processes, their integration and interaction. The earlier example of Mr B also illustrated the importance of individual cognitive functions in daily living, when loss of a single function such as calculation could lead to inability to maintain a job.

Why knowledge of impairment is important

So far it has been established that knowledge of cognitive processes is important in the analysis of occupational performance and the diagnosis of occupational difficulties (activity limitations and participation restrictions). But it is also important for occupational therapists to go further and be able to differentiate the relative contributions of different cognitive *impairments* in any given occupational dysfunction.

In the case of Mr B, his problems with completing complex tasks could have one or several causative factors:

1. Difficulties with recall might prevent him from remembering a set of instructions.
2. Problem-solving deficits might result in inability to apply rules to novel problems.
3. Lack of drive might mean he is readily discouraged from attempting something which appears difficult.

Knowledge of the possible sources of difficulty enables the therapist to identify which aspects of cognition need assessing, and how to decide upon the best treatment for this dysfunction. If Mr B's difficulty was arising predominantly from his poor recall, then provision of written instructions would enable him to succeed. But if the major difficulty was his problem-solving deficit, it would require treatment that enabled him to learn rules and practise their application in a graded programme of tasks that gradually increased in complexity.

Hence, one activity limitation could have several possible causes, and require a different treatment approach depending upon those causes. Selection of treatment without knowledge of cognition, careful occupational analysis and assessment of impairments would result in an unsuccessful outcome.

Putting knowledge and frameworks together

Frameworks such as the ICF and the OTPF provide us with tools to analyse human function, activities and the influence of environment and other contexts upon occupational performance. Skills of activity and occupational analysis provide the means to identify the components of human performance and the demands of the activities humans engage in. Neuropsychological theories, case studies and research methodology provide an understanding of cognitive

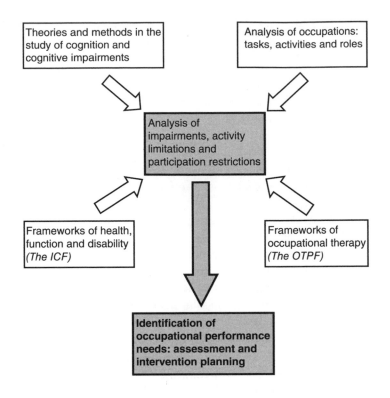

Fig. 1.6 Summary of the components of cognitive rehabilitation.

systems and their underlying processes. Neuropsychological tests provide health professionals with tools to measure impairments and a basis upon which to develop functional assessments.

When cognitive impairments occur as a result of trauma or disease, the knowledge, skills and tools of neuropsychology may act in combination with frameworks (which help us to structure and organise information) to provide a means to:

- Consider the possible nature of cognitive impairments from the location and extent of brain damage
- Screen, or specifically test for cognitive impairments
- Identify and analyse the cognitive components of activities and occupations
- Analyse and assess activity limitations and participation restrictions
- Consider and select effective treatment methods and strategies
- Determine the outcomes of intervention
- Consider the individual's longer-term needs

Figure 1.6 illustrates the contribution of knowledge and frameworks to the process of rehabilitation in which occupational therapists are engaged.

Summary

1. Cognitive deficits impact upon every aspect of life and can create difficulties in all areas of occupation. Because of the central role of cognition in human functioning, occupational therapists must have an understanding of cognition, and how cognitive abilities contribute to occupational performance.
2. The World Health Organisation has produced a framework of health and health-related states (WHO, 2001) that can be used to organise, define and examine the relationships between all areas and levels of human functioning. This includes cognitive functions, their associated body structures and their relationship to human activities and participation.
3. The concepts incorporated within the ICF make it complementary to and compatible with the OTPF (AOTA, 2001). This is a professional framework that guides occupational therapists in their analysis and understanding of human occupation and occupational performance difficulties.
4. Together with knowledge of cognition and cognitive impairments, these frameworks can be applied within the clinical reasoning process to guide comprehensive analysis of occupational performance needs and deficits. This in turn facilitates appropriate and effective assessment of cognitive deficits, and intervention planning.

2 Identifying and Assessing Cognitive Impairments

Introduction to assessment frameworks

Assessment is a fundamental component of any therapeutic inter-action between a health professional and client, and is considered the starting point of occupational therapy intervention. It requires the gathering together of information, identification of problems and measurement of the extent of their impact upon the individual within his or her particular life contexts (see Figure 2.1). Assessment initiates, but also takes place throughout the occupational therapy process, and is used to identify the client's strengths as well as areas of difficulty.

This chapter will consider the stages and components of the assessment process, and explore the factors the occupational therapist must consider in order to conduct thorough, timely and appropriate assessment that is of benefit to the client and facilitates effective rehabilitation.

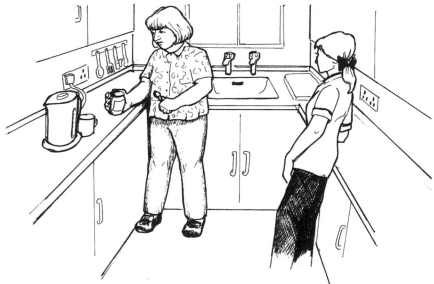

Fig. 2.1 Assessment identifies areas of ability as well as difficulty.

The OTPF organises categories of information geared to the priorities and concerns of the profession and reflects the relationship of performance skills to occupations and activities. This guides the therapist as to what information might be elicited through verbal communication (occupational history, needs etc.), and what is more suitably assessed through observation (occupational performance and performance skills). The ICF on the other hand, provides a comprehensive set of activity domains without differentiating between them in terms of occupational meaning and without indicating how they are most effectively assessed.

It is most helpful for the occupational therapist in practice to work with an occupational framework that incorporates and relates to the ICF framework. This ensures consistency of terminology and concepts whilst also adhering to the priorities and occupational focus of the profession. Figure 2.2 illustrates the relationship

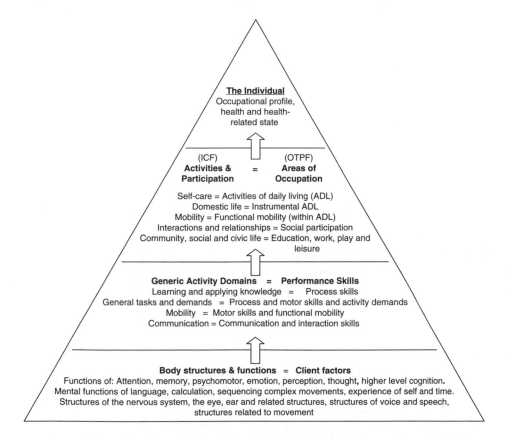

Fig. 2.2 Hierarchy of performance: the relationship between components of cognitive function, activity and occupation indicating the equivalence of the ICF and the OTPF.

of the components of each framework, in which each successive level of function is achieved through the effective operation of the levels beneath. These two frameworks are useful in everyday practice to provide comprehensive checklists, ensuring that nothing of relevance is omitted from the assessment process. They also serve to clarify the focus of assessment and help in the selection of appropriate methods and tools.

Initial assessment

The commonest methods for gathering initial information about a client are by interview and observation. Initial assessments are exploratory for both the therapist and the client. A checklist of basic information and a protocol of short tasks to enable preliminary observation of performance will often be sufficient to make a start on formulating further screening and assessment needs.

A standard checklist and protocol grounded in a clear theoretical framework is preferable to something developed ad hoc or 'in-house'. Using a published, accepted framework that is familiar within and between professions can facilitate good practice. Interprofessional understanding is enhanced if a framework incorporates all aspects and levels of function, and the concepts are understood by all. Hence, if an area of concern is identified at initial assessment, all members of the team will be able to locate this within the wider health context of the client and understand its relevance.

For multidisciplinary teams, assessment tools based upon or related to a generic health framework such as the ICF will facilitate interprofessional communication and clarity of terms and definitions. The use of uniform concepts and terminology may also reduce the frequency or necessity professionals often feel to repeat questions or basic procedures that colleagues have already performed.

As with any assessment process, it is important to prepare the client, oneself and the environment, and at the outset provide appropriate introductions and explanation of the purpose of the session. It is of particular importance to:

1. Obtain prior information – for example the client's first language and cultural background; family relationships; educational background and interests; hand dominance; history of the injury/illness and its management to date. Establish the client's current understanding of his health condition.

2. Arrange the environment – minimise distractions; ensure comfort, privacy, visibility and safe positioning.
3. Exclude confounding factors – drowsy from medication, infection, pain, constipation, check vision (glasses?), hearing (aid?), communication aids needed?
4. Consider the client's ability to cope – can the client sustain attention or cope with the demands of the process, will it need to be broken down into a series of shorter sessions, will rest breaks be needed?
5. Establish if any sensorimotor, visual or communication impairments are present. Assessment results from other health professionals are important sources of information. Often all members of the multidisciplinary team are concurrently involved in establishing the presence and extent of such impairments; therefore close cooperation and communication is essential.
6. Observe any declared precautions or contraindications – instructions such as 'nil by mouth', or manual handling directives could directly impact upon the occupational therapy assessment. Similarly, if a client is catheterised or fitted with other medical or surgical equipment, procedures may have to be modified to take these into account.

Making a start: initial interviews

Interviews serve many purposes: helping to establish the basis of the therapist–client relationship; gaining background information; identifying the most effective methods of communication with the client; starting to determine the client's problems, their goals and expectations, and the therapist's role in realising these.

Occupational therapy models and frameworks contribute to the construction of standardised interview tools. Instruments such as the Occupational Circumstances Assessment–Interview Rating Scale (OCAIRS, Hagland et al., 2001) and the Canadian Occupational Performance Measure (COPM, Law et al., 1998) explore in detail a person's occupational history, values and concerns. Such instruments require a certain level of functioning for the client to engage with them, not least, receptive and expressive communication skills, attention, concentration, memory, a certain level of fatigue resistance and a realistic appreciation of their own capacity and performance (insight).

Whilst such tools become useful in time, it is not advisable to introduce them before the client's ability to cope with them has been determined. Eventually, a tool such as the COPM (Law et al.,

1998) would be useful for goal setting and measuring progress with the client. It is both an assessment and an outcome measure that can be administered before, during and at the conclusion of treatment. This enables the client to determine goals jointly with the therapist, and evaluate their own progress through therapy. The use of standardised instruments will be considered later in this chapter.

Making a start: initial observations

Observation is the other principal way in which information is gathered to help inform the assessment process. When carried out informally, observations are rife with the potential for subjective interpretation and misleading inferences about what is observed. However, initial observations are informal procedures often undertaken during or alongside initial interviews.

Difficulties with task execution can arise for any number of reasons. Proper preparation of the client and the environment as described above can minimise and help to discount possible confounding factors. For example, if a client is asked to reach for a glass and take a drink of water from it, he may experience difficulty if he normally uses a hearing aid but is without it on this occasion. If the therapist is unaware of this sensory impairment she may observe a delay in task initiation and query receptive aphasia, visual-perceptual impairment or apraxia. Apparent difficulty with following instructions may have nothing to do with cognitive impairment but everything to do with the absence of everyday aids.

Initial observations should incorporate basic, short-term and familiar tasks. As a general rule, complicated and novel tasks make greater cognitive demands and could be beyond the abilities of a client; therefore there would be little benefit to either client or therapist in attempting these. Tasks that are useful in initial observation include those that can be naturally integrated into the assessment situation. The demands of the task are more likely to be appropriate to context, and this helps to avoid artificial procedures that may have no occupational meaning to the client, or whose function might not be understood.

Selection of suitable tasks to be performed during initial assessment will be guided by the client's level of functioning, the environment, and the range of cognitive demands the tasks make. The therapist makes use of occupational theory, activity analysis and knowledge of cognition in this process. Depending upon the environment and context (whether the assessment is taking place on a hospital ward, in a therapy department, or in the client's own home), a range of tasks need to be used which collectively make demands of all the elements of cognition. Visual perception, spatial abilities, attention, memory, purposeful movement and executive functions should all be assessed to some degree.

It is not possible to select tasks that will enable each component of cognition to be assessed in isolation. Even basic tasks have multiple cognitive components. The therapist should use tasks that are simple so that where possible each makes demands of one cognitive component more than others. Breaking one task down into component stages can achieve the same effect.

Having a selection of everyday items on a table in front of the client will enable the therapist to make a variety of cognitive demands through task selection. For example, items might include: magazines, pen and paper, water jug and glass, and a comb. These could be used to ask the client to:

- Point to an object: demanding visual perception (figure ground) and object recognition
- Pick up the object and move it to another position: demanding spatial abilities
- Use or mimic the use of the object: demanding object recognition and praxis
- Use two related objects (for example pour water into the glass); demanding all of the above, plus motor planning and sequencing, judgement and prediction

Note how this sequence of demands is organised so that the most simple comes first, and each task builds upon the successful completion of the others. Any difficulties with execution of the tasks should be recorded as observed. It is often tempting for a therapist to make inferences about the observation (Mr X could not reach for the glass because . . .), but this should be avoided. This is because:

1. There is insufficient information at this stage about the extent and nature of the client's impairments to make such inferences.
2. Informal procedures tend to vary between therapists and environments and so the client's performance may be influenced by factors other than his/her own impairments.

Accurate recording of observations is underpinned by the skill of activity analysis. The *form* of an occupation refers to how it is carried out (Hocking, 2001). An occupational therapist must have knowledge of the performance demands and performance components of an activity in order to observe its form as carried out by the client, and accurately record those aspects that cause difficulty. This includes not only the client's performance skills, but also any aspects of the environment that might be supporting or hindering his performance.

Initial observation is invaluable to screen in an informal way for activity limitations that may be occurring because of cognitive deficits. As emphasised above, one can only describe performance difficulties from such observations, not infer causation. Therefore initial observation can serve two purposes:

1. Observing the performance of activities may help to indicate the integrity or impairment of component body functions and structures.
2. Observing performance of basic activities will aid prediction of limitations in other areas of occupation and guide decisions on further assessment.

The outcome of initial assessment

Initial assessment should result in the acquisition of basic occupational information and an outline of occupational performance strengths and difficulties. The assessment should record the nature and extent of any observed disruption to task performance, and also note those elements of the task performed effectively.

Further formal screening and assessment may be necessary to fully explore the client's occupational performance and determine the impact of cognitive impairments more accurately. In some cases, an initial assessment reveals no apparent difficulties with task performance, but as the client progresses and resumes more complex occupational roles, impairments may become apparent, and the expected level of occupational performance is not achieved. Occasionally impairment may be highly specific and only seen in particular circumstances.

Comprehensive assessment

Approaches to assessment: occupation or impairment focused?

Decisions about the assessment of clients centre around the relationship between occupational performance, environmental factors (context) and underlying performance components (performance skills, body structures and body functions). The relevant issues are encompassed in the consideration of whether assessment should be 'top-down' or 'bottom-up', and are explored by Hocking (2001).

Top-down assessment assumes that occupational performance is the primary measure of a person's ability to function successfully within his environment. All elements, both external to and within the individual (roles, relationships, health, occupational identity, personal needs and priorities, environment), contribute to occupational performance. Assessment is occupationally focused, incorporating consideration of all these elements.

Bottom-up assessment is based upon the premise that the underlying performance components are key to successful occupational performance. Assessment and treatment of impairments will lead to the correction of occupational performance deficits and there is a direct relationship between impairment and function. Assessment is impairment focused.

A professional consensus is emerging that top-down or occupationally based assessments are most appropriate to the tenets and goals of occupational therapy. Evidence increasingly supports the view that impairments of body structure or function do not always equate directly with a given degree of occupational performance deficit, and impairment-level assessments cannot be relied upon alone to predict functional problems (Hocking, 2001).

The advantages of an occupational or top-down approach are:

- The client's experience of assessment is meaningful and is seen to relate directly to his/her occupational needs (see Figure 2.3).
- The relationship between assessment and interventions is clear.
- The occupational focus encourages the client's motivation and active participation.
- Assessment tools are more likely to hold value for use as outcome measures because of their functional content.

Occupation-focused assessment seeks to understand the nature and extent of a client's difficulties from his own perspective, taking into account occupational history, the person's role and responsibilities within the family and wider society, the activities that are necessary and appropriate in his everyday life, what is meaningful to him and what he wants and needs to achieve optimal occupational performance. Occupational assessment

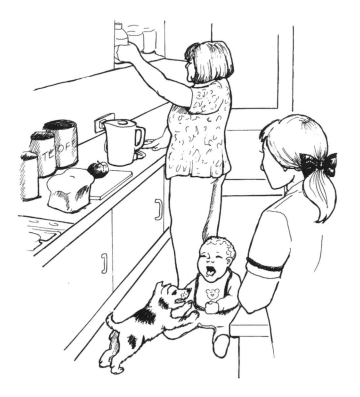

Fig. 2.3 Occupational assessment relates directly to occupational need.

incorporates both qualitative and quantitative elements; hearing the client's narrative, values and concerns, and observing and measuring functional abilities during activity.

Occupational therapists need to commence the assessment process from an occupational perspective. Appropriate interventions cannot be planned unless there is a thorough knowledge of the activities and occupations the client needs and wants to perform, an understanding of the contexts within which this person lives, or knowledge of basic cognitive abilities required for the performance of activities. Occupation-focused assessment enables the identification of overall goals, and delineates areas of function that are a priority, whether that means independence in self-care, the ability to manage a home, re-acquisition of work skills or improving general task skills across multiple areas of activity.

Impairment-level assessments continue to have an important role within cognitive rehabilitation. They should supplement and complement occupational assessments when:

- Deficits in cognitive performance components are suspected and need to be confirmed.
- Cognitive deficits are identified and their effects need to be fully ascertained.
- A client is in a low arousal state and occupational performance is severely restricted.

Impairment-level assessments can also be used to track any reduction in deficits that occurs as a result of recovery, or to identify that recovery is not occurring. Decisions to change treatment approaches from restorative to adaptive or compensatory can be supported by evidence from such assessments. For example, repeating a table-top assessment for visual neglect may show no improvement in this impairment, and a decision may be made to teach the client to scan visually during activities, to compensate for this persisting problem. An activities of daily living (ADL) assessment may show occupational improvement as a consequence.

The hierarchy of performance in Figure 2.2 illustrated the relationship of underlying components of human function to the occupational nature of the individual. It identified the equivalence of an occupational framework (OTPF) with the World Health Organisation's framework of health (ICF). It is also possible to locate assessment approaches within this hierarchy:

- Impairment-level assessments address functions at the level of client factors and performance skills – the base levels of the pyramid.
- Occupational assessments consider activity performance within areas of occupation – the higher levels of the pyramid.

The nature and content of any given assessment tool can be used to locate it within this hierarchy, helping to ascertain its value and appropriateness within the assessment process, and its relationship to other assessments. For example, the Rivermead Perceptual Assessment Battery (RPAB) (Whiting *et al.*, 1985) is a test which screens for perceptual deficits using a series of table-top tasks. It does not utilise familiar everyday activities, and is conducted in a standardised way intended to be the same for every client. It does not seek to measure performance of daily living activities, nor the client's ability to interact with the environment. The RPAB is an assessment of impairment. Within an occupational therapy assessment process, this tool would contribute valuable diagnostic information for the presence of perceptual deficits, indicating why a daily activity might create problems for a client. The results could guide the selection of adaptive strategies that might help to overcome these problems. The assessment could not provide a measure of occupational ability, nor predict a client's performance of familiar activities in a familiar setting. Hence, it would be effective at the level of client factors (body structures and function) and selected performance skills to screen for deficits that might warrant further investigation, or to track possible improvement. It could not reliably predict occupational performance.

Not all assessments fit neatly into specific levels of the hierarchy. Some standardised screening tools utilise activities to assess for discrete cognitive deficits, therefore serving a dual purpose of measuring aspects of activity performance as well as identifying underlying impairments. The Structured Observational Test of Function (Laver & Powell, 1995), and the Assessment of Motor and Process Skills (Fisher, 1997) assess both performance of activities and underlying performance skills. As such they can offer measures of occupational performance as well as identifying and measuring underlying impairments. These types of assessment may help to reduce the overall number of assessments a client is subjected to.

A thorough cognitive assessment process will incorporate a range of procedures and tools that address all levels of function relevant to each client's occupational needs: occupational performance, activity and task performance, cognitive performance skills and related client factors. Throughout the assessment process it is essential that the therapist utilises clinical reasoning to select the most appropriate tools for a given client and situation.

Ensuring that assessment is robust

Throughout the occupational therapy process, informal observation and interviews are two methods of information gathering that have an important role. Observing the client in his usual setting and while undertaking his usual daily routine can yield valuable insights into functional difficulties. Discussions with the client, his family and relevant others can provide illuminating information about context-specific behaviour and persisting or emerging areas of difficulty, as rehabilitation and resettlement progress.

We have considered the choice between occupationally-focused assessments and impairment-focused assessments. The second issue is how to decide upon the most appropriate method and tool. A number of factors must be taken into account:

- Appropriateness of standardised assessment
- Availability of suitable assessments
  - For the client
  - For the setting
  - In relation to the therapist's experience and knowledge

- Sensitivity, responsiveness and metric properties of the assessment
- Validity of the information collected and the reliability of the method used

All of the above factors have received considerable attention in the rehabilitation literature. Clive-Lowe (1996) outlined the importance of standardised assessment practices for occupational therapists, not just to ensure accurate assessment of individual clients, but also to contribute to the evidence base for practice, enhance service cost-effectiveness and enable accurate clinical audit. Hobart *et al.* (1996) and Wade (2004) emphasised the importance of standardisation to good clinical practice, and discussed the meaning of properties such as reliability, validity, sensitivity and responsiveness. Salter *et al.* considered selection issues in relation to outcome measures for stroke, relating these to the ICF components of body functions (assessment of impairment) (2005a), activity limitations (2005b) and participation restrictions (2005c). These papers collectively provide a comprehensive overview of factors important in the selection of measurement tools, applicable to cognitive rehabilitation as well as to neurological rehabilitation generally.

The focus of and priorities for assessment will be driven by multiple factors, in addition to the client's occupational needs and deficits, for example the role of the service provider and the therapist's work remit within it (acute rehabilitation, community support, respite care, vocational rehabilitation). Government initiatives, policies and guidelines may provide key directives for service priorities. Staff and other resource availability may determine which aspects of assessment are followed through, and which are referred on to other agencies.

Whatever the setting, the therapist must select and use robust assessment tools in an appropriate and timely way, that provide information of value to the client, therapist and other members of the multidisciplinary team. Figure 2.4 summarises the assessment

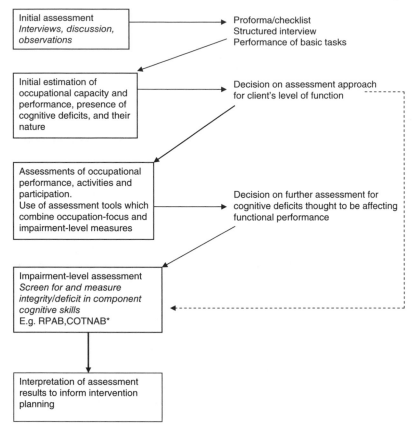

Fig. 2.4 The process of selecting assessments.

* Please refer to the key abbreviations given in the introduction to Part 2 (p. 59)

process, identifying the points at which various types of assessment should be considered.

Which assessment when?

The diagram in Figure 2.4 suggests that the decision-making process and the order in which types of assessments are used, is linear. The dotted line indicates that this may not always be the case. Occupation and impairment-level assessments may be carried out in parallel, or a client's deficits may be such that some tools such as occupational profiling and goal setting cannot be used prior to functional assessment. Impairments in higher level executive functions may limit the validity of client-centred tools such as the COPM because these functions are essential for the findings of the tool to be valid and reliable; the client needs to be able to appraise his situation. Deficits in global cognitive

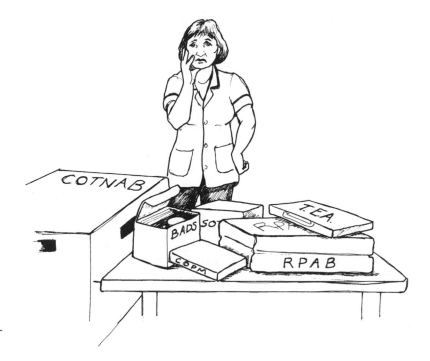

Fig. 2.5 Which assessment, when?

functions such as attention or memory will limit the client's participation in most activities, and so some assessments may have to be completed over several sessions, or a standardised tool may not be viable because a client cannot comply with the behavioural demands it makes.

The perfect assessment tool does not exist, neither does the perfect assessment protocol. The therapist must use clinical reasoning, guided by a series of key questions, to arrive at the most suitable choice of assessment methods and tools, for each client (see Figure 2.5).

Selecting the most suitable assessment

A first question is whether assessment should be occupationally focused or directed at the impairment level. Interview or observation of functional performance requires an occupationally-focused assessment (of participation, activity and task performance), whereas observation, diagnosis and measurement of discrete cognitive deficits will require impairment-level assessment. It should be remembered that some assessment tools may do both.

Should an assessment be standardised or non-standardised? A standardised measure is best if you are:

- Seeking a measure of capacity (you want to know the best possible level of ability in a standard environment) or of performance (you want to know how the client will be able to perform in his own environment)
- Intending to repeat this assessment to monitor progress, or to use it as an outcome measure
- Using results of the assessment to contribute to service evaluation/clinical research
- Predicting function in another area of activity (the assessment must have undergone research which shows its results are valid for this purpose)

A non-standardised measure will be suitable if you are:

- Seeking to solve a problem specific to this client's context
- Measuring performance, not capacity
- Unable to match the client to the criteria for a standardised assessment
- Unable to find a standardised assessment for your specific purpose

Considerations of the client's fitness to participate in the selected assessment

It is important to determine whether a client fits the criteria for use of a particular assessment – has it been validated for this clinical population/age group/culture? For example, some assessments may assess for cognitive impairments, but only for people with stroke, and some may exclude certain age groups.

Other considerations include whether any pre- or co-morbid factors exclude your client from an assessment, for example epilepsy or a history of aggression. Are there any contraindications to its use? Can the client cope with the procedural and performance demands of undergoing this assessment? Are there any communication problems, physical limitations, or sensory impairments?

Considerations for the therapist when selecting an assessment

It is important to be familiar with the structure and properties of a number of standardised occupation-focused and impairment-level assessments, to assist with the selection of appropriate tools.

- Is training necessary for the reliable and valid administration of this assessment?
- If you are proposing to use only a subsection of this assessment, will this affect its validity and reliability?
- If the client shows improvement on an assessment over time, is there a possibility that this is because they are learning how to do the assessment, rather than because their cognitive performance skills are actually improving?

Summary

1. The Occupational Therapy Practice Framework (AOTA, 2002) incorporates all elements of the ICF (WHO, 2001), enabling the occupational therapist to use it as a guiding framework in the assessment of cognitive impairments and their impact upon occupational performance.

2. Informal interview and task observations are useful to assist in the initial assessment of a client before more comprehensive and formal assessments are undertaken. Care must be taken in the preparation of the client, selection of suitable tasks and interpretation of findings at this stage.

3. Comprehensive assessment of the client incorporates both occupation-focused and impairment-level approaches. Occupational or top-down assessments should be considered as primary tools. These are most appropriate to the tenets and goals of occupational therapy. Impairment-level or bottom-up assessments are essential for investigating underlying cognitive deficits in detail, and to aid decision making in relation to treatment approaches and methods.

4. The assessment process must be robust. This is dependent upon the application of sound clinical reasoning within a clear assessment procedure. Many factors must be taken into account when deciding upon assessment tools; these relate to the client, the service setting, the availability and utility of assessment tools, and their properties. Reliability, the validity of the findings and the uses to which the results are put, should be included.

3 Intervention for Cognitive Impairments

Occupational therapists draw upon theory, evidence, expert opinion and the tenets of the profession, to seek the best possible outcomes for their clients. Cerebral injuries often result in cognitive deficits that do not completely resolve, and the therapist must work to minimise the effects of these deficits upon the individual, their occupational performance, roles and life in general.

Evidence for the effectiveness of particular interventions is debatable. The occupational therapist uses sound clinical reasoning in the selection and application of interventions, considering the theories and evidence upon which they are based. Just as assessment is an essential stage in planning interventions, so outcome measurement is also crucial to evaluate the impact and effect of interventions and enable professional practice to evolve and develop.

The aims of this chapter are to:

- Identify factors that will influence the rehabilitation process
- Introduce the performance objectives of occupational therapy intervention
- Discuss the selection and use of approaches in intervention
- Describe methods and techniques used in cognitive rehabilitation
- Consider parameters for evaluating the outcomes of intervention

Factors influencing the rehabilitation process

Teamworking

The overall goal of rehabilitation is jointly determined with other members of the multidisciplinary team. The team comprises other health and social care professionals, and most importantly the client and relevant others (see Figure 3.1). It may extend to incorporate support staff, residential institutions, voluntary helpers or employers, depending upon the situation and the client's needs. Effective rehabilitation and management requires the ability to formulate a clear plan of action and follow it through. Throughout the intervention process, this plan must be reviewed and the client's progress monitored, in consultation with the wider team. Decisions about the focus of intervention, the most effective methods to employ, intensity and frequency of treatment, and when to modify interventions, will all be influenced to some extent by the opinions of the team and the needs of the client's relevant others. Cognitive rehabilitation can be a long-term process and the team members are likely to change over time, as the client's needs change.

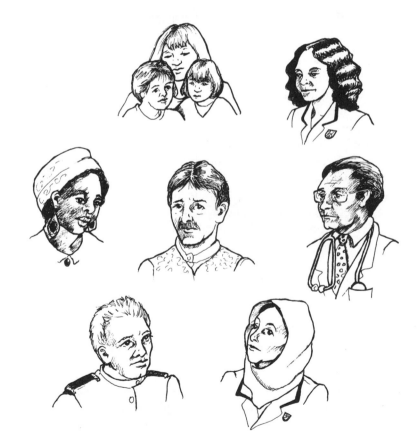

Fig. 3.1 The client is at the centre of the rehabilitation team.

Health and safety

When considering intervention, health and safety is a primary concern. It will determine whether an intervention is feasible, regardless of any potential therapeutic benefit or occupational priority. All health and social care professions encode safety concerns in their ethical and professional codes of conduct (see COT, 2005). The guidance for preparation for initial assessments given in Chapter 2 applies equally to intervention and treatment sessions, emphasising the safety of the client and the therapist. For people with cognitive deficits, the environment can present constant challenges. Disorientation arising from impaired memory, or underlying attentional problems, may give rise to risk in apparently low-risk situations. Lack of insight into their own health and abilities may lead clients to undertake activities beyond their capacity (for example a client may try to get out of bed unaided although only able to bear weight through one leg).

Metacognition: insight and self-awareness

When body structures or functions become damaged and impaired, treatment, recovery and rehabilitation require the active cooperation and participation of the individual. This is one of the central tenets of occupational therapy and rests upon the ability of the person to understand and engage with therapy. This ability stems from many intra-personal factors, two of which are the degree of insight a person has into his condition and the degree of self-awareness. Unlike damage to other body systems, when the brain sustains damage these functions may be directly impaired.

Metacognition is the term that encompasses the functions and processes of self-awareness and insight. Both derive from effective executive functioning (see Chapter 10). Metacognitive deficits may result in:

- Lack of knowledge of impairments
- Difficulty understanding the impact of impairments upon abilities and performance
- Inability to effectively direct and adjust thoughts and behaviours to solve problems or to form a realistic appreciation of a situation

Such deficits will have a major impact upon the effectiveness of rehabilitation and will influence the choice of treatment approaches and methods that might be used. When a client has full awareness of and insight into his deficits this can also impact upon his ability to engage with treatment. For example, being unable to remember the way from one place to another (topographical disorientation), or to recognise familiar faces (prosopagnosia), can be distressing, frustrating and embarrassing (see Figure 3.2). Anxiety arising from these experiences may compound a client's difficulties, worsening performance or lowering motivation. It may further impair judgement and lead to poor decision making. Careful preparation, orientation of the client and attention to his safety and comfort, will contribute to a sense of emotional security and confidence, and support his ability to engage with interventions.

Time course and pattern of recovery

There are generally recognised timeframes for the different stages and processes of recovery following brain injury. Service provision and therapeutic interventions should match the client's needs and progress as closely as possible. Figure 3.3 illustrates the typical time course and stages in rehabilitation. Variations occur between individuals in the progress made and the services they may access,

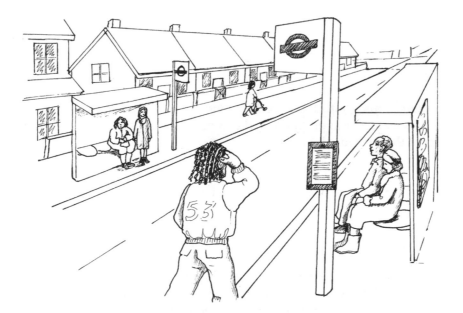

Fig. 3.2 Topographical disorientation can be distressing.

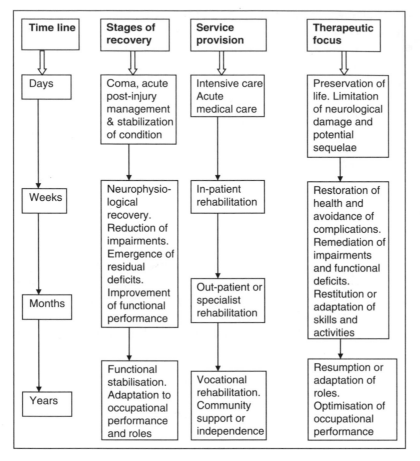

Fig. 3.3 The time course of recovery and rehabilitation.

as well as the eventual outcome of rehabilitation. The nature of therapeutic input must be appropriate to the stage of recovery and progression of the individual.

Performance objectives of occupational therapy

Occupational performance requires the effective use of perform-ance skills, organised into performance patterns, within areas of occupation (OTPF, AOTA, 2002). These patterns consist of habits, routines and roles. An effective programme of intervention incor-porates cognitive objectives to enable achievement of effective patterns that underpin the ultimate goal of successful occupa-tional performance. Objectives must incorporate the observable

Table 3.1 Performance objectives of occupational interventions.

Performance pattern	Cognitive performance objective	Characteristics of performance
Habits	Automatic execution of tasks	Consistent sequence of actions Consistent use of tools within a consistent environment
Routines	Performance of tasks in an established sequence Able to transfer performance to other similar environments	Logical order Context appropriate Time appropriate Transferable
Roles	Performance of activities incorporating a variety of tasks, in variable contexts	Consistent and appropriate execution of tasks and activities in sequence and according to context Transferable and generalisable to a range of environments Able to adapt in novel situations

and measurable characteristics of each performance pattern, so that progress towards them can be monitored and evaluated. The objectives for any given goal will mark the client's progress and form the framework for the intervention programme. Table 3.1 identifies key objectives of cognitive interventions, together with the performance characteristics that indicate their successful achievement.

Table 3.1 illustrates that each level of performance (habit, routine, or role; AOTA, 2002) builds upon the preceding one, and with each successive level, the complexity of demands upon cognition increases. Habitual performance is characterised by automatic behaviours. Routines require a combination of automaticity with transferability. Role performance requires the ability to apply a range of strategies in varying contexts with a range of demands. Each level makes increasing demands upon problem solving and other executive functions. Intervention should address the level of performance at which the client begins to exhibit difficulty. For example, seeking to remediate the performance of routines if habits are not established will impose demands upon the client in excess of abilities. This will result at best in unsuccessful intervention, and at worst in non-cooperation and disengagement of the client.

Selecting and using therapeutic approaches

What is an approach?

The professional taxonomy of occupational therapy can be confusing. Some terms are used interchangeably in the published literature. For example, the ICF is referred to in this book, and by the World Health Organisation (Dahl, 2001; WHO, 2001) as a framework. It is referred to by the College of Occupational Therapists as both a framework and a model (COT, 2004) and by some authors (for example Bilbao *et al.*, 2003) as a model. Within the field of cognitive rehabilitation, the terms 'approach' and 'model' also seem to be used interchangeably (see Lee *et al.*, 2001).

In brief, models and frameworks form bases upon which to organise and prioritise information about a client and identify treatment needs, as we have seen in Chapter 2. The term 'approach' concerns how a model or framework is put into operation in interventions. An approach usually derives from one or more related theories and specifies how problems (impairments, performance deficits) should be dealt with. Quite often, a therapist will select and use several approaches with a client in order to address a range of problems, or to meet needs as they change over time.

Within cognitive rehabilitation, approaches to intervention have traditionally fallen into one of two categories: *remedial* and *adaptive*. Occupational therapists utilise both, but are concerned with the ability of the client to perform within their own life and environmental contexts. This has led to the formulation of a third, *functional*, approach.

The remedial approach

The remedial approach aims to restore and improve impaired functions by supporting and facilitating the brain's capacity for recovery and plasticity. This approach is derived from theories of recovery from cerebral injury. It assumes a capacity for recovery of functions, through such processes as axonal sprouting, synaptic plasticity and reorganisation of function in which undamaged areas of the brain take over functions of damaged areas. Treatment methods aimed at improving specific impairments (for example memory training, table-top perceptual exercises) are hypothesised to result in improvement of these components, and this in turn will lead to improvement in functional performance.

The adaptive approach

This approach recognises that cognitive impairments frequently persist to some degree following cerebral injury, based upon the premise that recovery within the central nervous system is limited. The focus is upon optimising remaining functions, and utilising the person's capacity for learning new strategies and techniques to overcome difficulties. This also incorporates manipulation of the environment to meet the person's needs. Improvement in functional abilities is sought through the use of strategies and techniques to compensate for impairments. Treatment methods utilise theories of learning, and may involve adaptation of activities or of the environment to compensate for persisting limitations, and optimise independence. In the case of a person with persistent deficits of figure-ground discrimination (see Chapter 5), the use of bright colours to differentiate crockery would help to locate and identify these items in a cluttered kitchen.

Which approach, when?

It is an ethical duty of all health services to seek the best outcome for any client. The major objective of all interventions is to enable the client to achieve their optimal level of independent functioning in all areas of life, with the best possible health status. Remediation is always the primary approach, congruent with this aim of recovery and restitution of impaired body structures and functions.

Adaptation can be used either as part of an overall remediation programme, or as the predominant approach if a client has reached a plateau in intrinsic recovery and shows no signs of any further progress. Adapting an activity to reduce its cognitive demands upon an individual may be important in the early stages of rehabilitation. As the client's performance improves, the adaptation may be removed to increase the challenge of the activity and bring the client's performance to within normal parameters.

In this way, adaptation is used as a *technique* to grade intervention, within a remedial approach.

Adaptation as an approach may involve adapting the client's environment in preparation for their return home, or teaching the use of equipment to compensate for permanent impairments. For example, in the case of memory impairment, a client may use a written timetable or reminders to support daily routines.

A third way – the functional approach

Realistically, a therapist will rarely use one approach to the total exclusion of another. The combination of approaches and techniques employed within a rehabilitation programme will derive from assessment and analysis of the client's strengths and difficulties and the nature of the pathology or damage he has sustained.

Lee *et al.* (2001) proposed a 'functional' model of cognitive rehabilitation, which argued that occupational therapy interventions are a balance between remedial and adaptive approaches. It is not possible to identify the degree of plasticity and potential for remediation within any one person's central nervous system. Rather than seeking to categorise whether a client has remedial potential or not at any given point in the rehabilitation process, the functional model supports the client-centred view, that performance is the outcome of interplay between external environmental factors and client-related factors. As such, any activity performed within a context will have both remedial and adaptive properties. The balance between remediation and adaptation comes from recognising and using each situation as therapeutically as possible, and accurately measuring the client's performance and progress.

Contextual factors facilitate or hinder performance. Evidence for this comes from research into memory and recall (see Chapter 8). Many occupational therapists see this in assessments of people with dementia; a person who is unable to locate items or sequence tasks in the unfamiliar surroundings of an ADL kitchen can undertake the same tasks without difficulty in his own home surroundings (see Figure 3.4). We take cues constantly from the environment in order to act appropriately and effectively. When cues are altered or absent, additional cognitive demands are placed upon us to solve problems, to locate, identify and learn the use of unfamiliar objects, or to apply prior knowledge to a new situation (transfer skills).

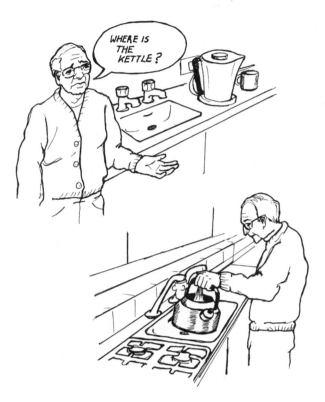

Fig. 3.4 A person may not recognise common items outside familiar contexts.

Knowledge about the role of context in performance enables the occupational therapist to manipulate activities and environments for remediation or adaptation. The functional approach recognises that basic cognitive processes are involved in every activity and situation; therefore, whether seeking remediation or adaptation, demands are made upon cognition in order to achieve learning and to carry out what has been learned in one or more situations. Regardless of approach, all therapeutic interventions require the client to learn, whether it is a case of relearning prior skills and activities, learning new ways to compensate for lost abilities, or learning new skills for the first time. Refer to Toglia (1991) for further reading on generalisation of treatment.

Methods and techniques in cognitive rehabilitation

A wide range of methods and techniques are utilised in cognitive rehabilitation. This section provides an overview and description of the main types. At the end of each chapter, from Chapters 5 to

10, suggestions are made for the specific application of methods and techniques, and for further reading of the evidence base.

Facilitators and barriers to learning

The ability to learn and acquire skills and competence is affected by both external and internal, or client-related, factors. Thorough assessment enables the therapist to identify these, and establish the starting point for intervention. Key factors include:

- Client related

    — Attentional level and distractibility
    — Behavioural difficulties
    — Sensory processing and perceptual difficulties
    — Fatigue and pain
    — Sensory or motor impairments
    — Literacy level
    — Language and communication skills
    — Cultural aspects of interaction with others and the environment
    — Values and goals

- External

    — Physical environment – noise, temperature, light, movement and clutter
    — Behaviour of the therapist
    — Presence or absence of significant others
    — Accessibility to comfort needs – toilet, fluids, food

It is important to recognise the role played by the family and wider social network of the client in a rehabilitation programme. The consequences of brain injury or disease can be devastating to family members, and have emotional, social and economic consequences for all. People are often highly motivated to do whatever possible to assist their loved one's recovery. The family and others may be the most valuable resource of all to the client and the therapist should always seek to engage their active participation. If a client is not an in-patient, he is likely to spend most of his time in his home environment, or perhaps vocational or educational settings. Significant others can be taught how to support, encourage and reinforce what is learned in intervention, or to continue a programme of activity with the client in his own context. In the case of a client returning home with persistent disabilities and dependence needs, the family will have care responsibilities and need preparation and support for these. Judgement is required as to the impact such roles might have upon family relationships, or the extent to which someone might feel able to manage certain tasks or behaviours, but the therapeutic potential is highly valuable and carries benefits for all.

Learning and behavioural methods

The environment can be used to influence behaviour, and to optimise learning. If a client's aggression appears to be made worse by stimuli such as sudden noises or movements, then the environment should be altered to minimise these, or prevent the client from being exposed to them. Similarly, if a client is distractible or has visual perception difficulties, a quiet, uncluttered room with minimal visual distractions will facilitate attention and reduce the visual processing demands of the environment.

Meaning and motivation derive from the client's engagement in goal setting. A client with limited insight and metacognitive abilities may be unable to identify or formulate long-term goals, may not see any need for them, and may have difficulty identifying progress towards them. Behavioural methods may be utilised in which desired behaviour is shaped by positive reinforcement or the gaining of meaningful rewards.

Behavioural methods may also be necessary for clients who exhibit behavioural sequelae associated with brain injury, such as disruption, aggression or disinhibition. Withholding rewards, ignoring undesirable behaviours and praising or rewarding appropriate behaviours, are some ways of utilising these methods. It is essential that all members of the rehabilitation team adopt the same methods and do so consistently, to ensure that they are effective.

Shaping

Shaping is a behavioural technique. It is used to encourage performance towards an end goal, when that end goal is not immediately achievable. In the early stages, any behaviour which approximates the desired performance is praised or otherwise rewarded, and so the client is encouraged towards behaving in that way. Once a component or level of behaviour has been achieved consistently, praise is no longer given, but is given if the next level of behaviour is achieved. Once the desired performance is fully achieved, praise is gradually reduced and stopped. This technique requires that the goal performance or behaviour is analysed and broken down into sequential stages. If several team members are involved in this intervention, all must know what the stages are, which stage the client has reached, and be agreed on the form of praise or reward to be given. Accurate record keeping and good communication are essential. Dysexecutive syndrome (see Chapter 10) can lead to impulsivity and inappropriate behaviour in social situations, such as the use of sexual innuendo or over affectionate advances to relative strangers. Prompt and frequent praise for acceptable and appropriate behaviour would provide the individual with positive attention and reward, reinforcing it over time.

Cueing

Cueing is a process of guiding and directing performance. If a person is unable to execute a task or activity from prior ability, or is learning a new skill, then guidance can be given as cues. It is important to use cues that are as simple as necessary for the person's level of function, and in the medium that can be most easily processed. Brain damage often results in difficulty processing large or abstract pieces of information and verbal cues should be suitably concise and simple. Cues can be visual (demonstration), verbal (spoken or written instructions), tactile (guiding or placing a body part), or environmental (for example, colour coding items or areas). They provide the client with information about what to do next in a sequence of actions and to improve quality of performance. Cues can be provided throughout a process, or only for parts that the person has difficulty with (see Figure 3.5). This technique is useful to grade activity demands as a person's performance improves. Frequent and simple cues provide maximum guidance and support in the early stages of practice, and can help to avoid failure. They can be increased in complexity and/ or decreased in frequency until the whole activity is performed without cues. This technique enables simultaneous treatment of more than one problem, for example whilst the person is learning to do a task, the form and content of the cues can be adjusted to make varying demands upon attention, sensory processing and

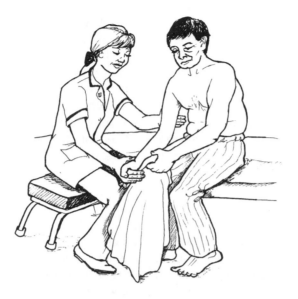

Fig. 3.5 Cueing is a process of guiding and directing performance.

memory. Cues are a useful indicator of progress for a client. The form, frequency and content of cues used in the same activity over time can be recorded to provide a record of performance, and serve as a measure of outcome.

Chaining

Chaining is a learning technique which can be applied either as forward chaining or backward chaining. The chosen task is broken down into stages. In forward chaining, the client completes the first stage of the task and the therapist completes the remainder. Once the client has mastered this stage, he/she goes on to complete both the first and second stage, and the therapist completes the remaining stages. Gradually, the client completes successive stages until he is undertaking the complete task. In backward chaining the reverse applies. The therapist completes all stages of the task except the last one, which the client completes. The therapist then completes all but the last two stages, which the client completes, and so on until he is undertaking the whole task. This latter method is useful because it gives the client the experience of completing a task, hence more satisfaction than the forward chaining method. This technique inherently grades a task in terms of duration, energy demands, complexity and information processing skills, gradually building the demands upon the person. Whole sequences of tasks and activities can be chained, and chaining can incorporate cueing to facilitate the gradual increase in a client's functional performance. Deficits of selective attention and distractibility (see Chapter 7) can prevent a person from completing tasks successfully, if at all. Backward chaining of routinely performed activities, such as making hot drinks, or getting dressed, is a useful form of grading the activity demands. In the early stages the goal is achieved with minimal opportunities for distraction, and the demands upon attention can be increased to facilitate improved performance over time.

Errorless learning

Errorless (or error-free) learning requires that the learner only experiences the correct way to undertake a task. The therapist provides instructions, cues or prompts such that no mistakes are made. This method is useful for people who have severe memory impairments or who are learning a task or activity that is to be used within one setting (not required to be transferable or generalisable), such as shaving every morning in the bathroom. Recall of previous performances will not contain erroneous information which might interfere with subsequent attempts. Demands upon problem solving and judgement are minimal as the environment and context of the task performance remains the same. The effectiveness of this method depends largely upon the repetitiveness of the whole task experience. Hence, transferability of the learning is not expected to occur.

Patterns of practice

Brain damage can result in permanent inability to problem solve, inability to transfer skills to other situations, or to develop them into generalised schemas, as discussed in Chapter 9. Even if high level cognitive functions are intact, the acquisition or re-acquisition of motor skills and task competence requires practice, and intervention programmes must incorporate practice schedules. The most commonly used types of practice schedule are *blocked practice* and *random practice*.

Blocked practice involves the repetition of the same sequence of actions repeatedly. Blocks of practice can be chained so that each element in a sequence is rehearsed repeatedly on its own before the whole is put together. Contextual interference is minimal in this situation, as the demands of the action or task remain the same each time. If using blocked practice to learn to throw and catch a ball, one element would be practised repeatedly, then the other, and only after acquisition of each element would the whole sequence of throwing followed by catching be put together. Random practice also involves repetition of the skill or task sequence, but with varying contextual demands, such as learning to catch and throw the ball in one sequence. The same schedules could be applied to putting a kettle on for tea; in blocked practice, each stage (picking up the kettle, filling it with water, placing it down and switching it on) would be rehearsed on its own repeatedly; in random practice the whole sequence would be performed at each repetition. Random practice increases the variability of demands upon performance, as there is increased contextual interference and the need to relate one stage or element to the next. In terms of learning, some evidence suggests that random practice leads to better retention and transferability of skills, but blocked practice improves performance during the process of acquisition (Flinn & Radomski, 2002). In terms of functional outcome, random practice might be considered more appropriate to the objectives and goals of occupational therapy, but clients with low level cognitive function may benefit more from blocked practice as it reduces cognitive demands during rehearsal, and may provide immediate experience of success. Varying practice schedules as a client progresses is another way of grading intervention.

Feedback and knowledge of results

Feedback and knowledge of results is essential to learning. We use *intrinsic* feedback, information derived via our senses, in the execution of all tasks and activities. We use the knowledge of results of our actions to evaluate their effectiveness, and feedback from our sensory systems to modify and refine our performance. *Extrinsic* feedback is that provided by others, again as a means of giving knowledge of results, or to monitor performance as it progresses. An important element of feedback and knowledge of results is the emotional element. The type of feedback we receive from others and from knowledge of results can provide satisfaction, reward and motivation, or disappointment and disinterest (see Figure 3.6). Feedback is therefore an important therapeutic and learning tool, and is a prominent feature of behavioural methods. Feedback can be positive or negative, given immediately, delayed, at intervals during a process, or as a summary at completion. It may be used to highlight errors, draw attention to aspects of

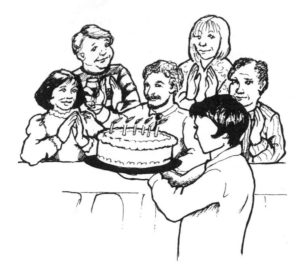

Fig. 3.6 Positive feedback from others can be a source of satisfaction and motivation.

performance, reinforce correct performance and highlight the relationship between actions and their consequences. How effectively a person learns may be determined by the type and pattern of feedback received, both in relation to the nature of the task, and in relation to his own personality and the cognitive deficits experienced. Positive verbal feedback given frequently may maintain attention and motivation, but if continued over time may lead to the person relying upon it rather than their own intrinsic systems. This may hinder learning. Feedback given during practice may distract and hinder performance for someone with attention deficits. Feedback given only in summary at the end of a task may be of limited value in the case of short-term memory problems. Again, this points to feedback as another tool for grading interventions. As a client progresses, feedback may be faded out to encourage consolidation of learning, reliance upon intrinsic feedback mechanisms and upon personal judgement. Alternatively, interim feedback may be a tactic to challenge attention and test distractibility.

Grading interventions

Grading is an important tool in the therapist's repertoire. As we have seen in the preceding section, behavioural, learning and teaching methods have inherent properties which allow grading to occur. The 'how', 'when' and 'what' of grading depends entirely upon the needs and progression of the individual client, and so there is no set formula or prescription. In addition to the specific aspects of intervention discussed above, the broader components of a programme or schedule should also be considered as a means to alter demands upon the individual, or adjust tasks and activities to their needs and capacities. These are:

- Time – the frequency and duration of sessions and activities can be increased or decreased to accommodate or challenge a person's energy levels, endurance and fatigue resistance.
- Complexity – contextual interference, environmental demands and the nature of tasks and activities all impose varying demands upon cognitive abilities, and can be manipulated to lessen or increase performance demands.
- Therapeutic use of self – the therapist's skills of communication and social skills mean that alongside specific techniques such as cueing and feedback, the use of verbal and non-verbal behaviour can be used to vary the therapeutic relationship as an intervention programme progresses. This might mean adjusting from a parental role to that of an equal participant in the rehabilitation process, or shifting decision taking from therapist to client as judgement and insight improve. Empowerment, personal responsibility, respect and choice are basic human rights. Brain damage results in deficits which frequently compromise these fundamental aspects of human existence, and restoring these are the most important, if rarely specified, goals of rehabilitation.

Evaluating the outcomes of interventions

Outcomes or effectiveness?

Just as it is important to identify the nature and type of a person's difficulties in order to plan interventions (assessment), so it is equally important to know the effects and consequences for the person of those interventions (evaluation of outcome). Outcome is perhaps a misnomer. It implies an end point and a conclusion, whereas the individual with brain damage continues to live with the impact of that damage upon their quality of life and that of those around them. Outcome measurement is a part of the intervention process which seeks to establish the effectiveness of the intervention, and not to draw a line under the client's progress. This is an important distinction to make, in order to avoid the implication that discharge from a programme of rehabilitation equates to the end of a client's recovery, or the end of potential for change. This discussion concerns the parameters for evaluating outcomes in terms of *effectiveness* of interventions, as well as the client's progress.

Evaluation for what purpose?

Evaluation is primarily viewed as a means to measure the client's progress. It is also a vital component in measuring service effectiveness. Every therapist has a duty to provide evidence of personal effectiveness, to contribute to the evidence base for service provision and utilise therapeutic approaches and methods that work. This derives from the ethical obligation to provide the best service to the client and provide best value to stakeholders in the service. Measurement of outcome specifically contributes to audit of service effectiveness and the development of evidence-based practice.

Evaluating the client's progress requires a comparison of performance against predetermined standards. These standards may derive from a range of sources: baseline measures derived from earlier assessments; normative population data; the client's own chosen goals; or the measurable objectives devised as part of the intervention plan.

Methods of evaluation

Reassessment and baseline measures

One of the most reliable ways to identify change in a client's abilities over time is to re-administer tests or assessments done previously. Assessments used in the early stages of intervention can be used again. This will provide reliable evidence of change if the instrument is standardised, but care must be exercised as to the purpose and validity of repeating an assessment. Occupational goals and objectives relate to functional performance, and while an assessment of impairment may show change in that impairment, this may not equate to improved functional performance, as was discussed in Chapter 2. For this reason, in terms of the client's progress there is less emphasis upon measurement of impairment at the end of intervention, and more use of functional outcome measures. Functional measures should be selected to address activity performance and provide information that is relevant to the client's current and future occupational performance needs.

From the service perspective, assessing impairments through-out a programme of intervention may provide useful evidence for the pattern or progression of recovery of underlying cognitive deficits. Such evidence, collected from many clients or even across services, could contribute to clinical decision making about when to apply particular approaches or techniques in the recovery process. Functional outcome measures provide information on the levels of independence and activity achieved during the rehabilitation process, and are key indicators of service outcome and effectiveness.

Comparison to normative data

This involves comparing the client's level and quality of function with population norms. For example, standardised tests of time taken to solve problems, or to don clothing, or of errors made in a particular task, can yield a measure of where a client is positioned within a distribution curve. Such information is rarely of value to a client unless there is a particular reason to know it, for example exploring suitability for a specific job in which performance times and accuracy had to fall within a certain normative range. Comparing client performance to normative data can be of value to services and individuals in researching the efficacy of specific interventions, or the extent to which particular cognitive deficits limit recovery.

Goal attainment

Degree of progression towards a goal can be measured objectively and subjectively. Objective measures, such as observations and standardised functional assessments provide external evidence as proof of goal achievement. Subjective measures include the client's own views and opinions of his progress. Together, these not only identify the degree of goal attainment, but can indicate the quality of the goal-setting process. An individual therapist or a service provider who finds that goals are persistently not achieved, or whose clients are not satisfied with their progress, might use this as evidence of a need to review the goal-setting process.

Objectives

Objectives are statements of achievement. They should be measurable, observable and specific, identifying the required components of successful performance. Written well and in sufficient detail, they form the framework for achievement of each goal within an intervention programme and are useful indicators of progress. For client, therapist and the service, they provide evidence of goal achievement, or the degree of progress a client is making towards a goal. They are sound and valid adjuncts to standardised outcome measures in providing evidence of client progression.

Summary

1. In conjunction with Chapters 1 and 2, this chapter has explored the occupational therapy process, with a specific focus upon intervention.

2. A practical approach is taken to intervention, focusing upon the work done with the client, rather than with relevant others. The first section considered factors that impinge upon the occupational therapy process and are likely to shape intervention beyond the needs and goals of the client and therapist. Team and service factors, recovery potential and the wider environmental context will influence the process. Objectives are important in the intervention process, both as markers for progress and for setting the basic structure for goal achievement. The ability to analyse and grade performance is essential for setting appropriate objectives, and the OTPF provides a useful framework.

3. Approaches to intervention are an important consideration. Remediation and adaptation form the two basic components, but a functional approach that incorporates both is most suited to the purposes of occupational therapy.

4. Learning is central to cognitive rehabilitation, whether the underlying approach has a stronger emphasis on remediation or adaptation. Many internal and external factors can act as barriers and facilitators to learning and must be considered in every intervention.

5. The family and significant others may play a pivotal role in meeting the rehabilitation and care needs of a client and are essential members of the team.

6. A range of intervention methods and techniques, derived from behavioural and learning theory, form the common components of intervention. Every person experiences the consequences of brain injury differently, and the particular mix of methods and techniques will reflect each person's needs.

Consistency of approach and communication between team members, particularly in the use of behavioural methods, is important. Grading is an inherent part of many techniques, but general aspects of intervention, the environment and the therapist's behaviour, are also useful tools.

7. Evaluating the outcomes of intervention is essential for all those involved. The key parameters for selecting and using different types of measures relate to the needs of the client, the therapist and the service. The use of functional measures enables evaluation of the client's progress and provides data on service outcomes. It is important to emphasise that discharge from a particular service or intervention programme does not mark the end of rehabilitation for the client, but is part of an ongoing process in which change will continue to occur.

Part 2 Components and Disorders of Cognition

In a person with brain damage, it is easy to recognise the physical changes which affect function. When there is impairment of cognition, the effects are often hidden and they offer barriers to physical rehabilitation. This section of the book was written to enable occupational therapists to develop an understanding of normal cognition in order to predict the effects of cognitive impairments in people with brain damage and to develop strategies to overcome them.

Part 2 begins with a summary of the methods and techniques used in the study of cognition. An overview of the structure and function of the brain is included. Next, each of the components of the cognitive system, together with their associated disorders, is presented in separate chapters. The adoption of this approach will enable the reader to appreciate the role in everyday living for each area of cognition. Accounts of classical experimental studies are given, often with a historical perspective. It is hoped that this will encourage the reader to seek out further literature in neuropsychology.

The inclusion of case studies aims to link the theory in psychology to the practice of occupational therapy. Suggestions for assessment and intervention for each component of cognition are presented at the end of each chapter.

Standardised tests suitable for the assessment of cognition are quoted by initials. The full titles are given below:

AMPS:	Assessment of Motor and Process Skills
BADS:	Behavioural Assessment of Dysexecutive Syndrome
BIT:	Behavioural Inattention Test
COTNAB:	Chessington Occupational Therapy Neurological Assessment Battery
LOTCA:	Lowenstein Occupational Therapy Cognitive Assessment
RPAB:	Rivermead Perceptual Assessment Battery
RBMT:	Rivermead Behavioural Memory Test
TEA:	Test of Everyday Attention

4 Cognition: Methods and Processes

What is cognition?

The information entering the brain from the environment is constantly changing. We adapt to these changes and respond to them by modifying our actions and behaviour. New information entering the system is organised, classified and stored for future use. Stored knowledge from our experience is retrieved and integrated with the current input. Plans for future action and behaviour are retrieved and activated at the right time and place. Cognition is all the mental processes in the brain concerned with this acquisition and use of knowledge.

The early stage in the processing of sensory information is perception, sometimes defined as 'making sense of the senses'. Perception organises sensory information from the environment into a meaningful whole. All the senses: vision, sound, touch, pain and proprioception, pick up information from the world around us, and from inside the body. The brain transforms all this input into our immediate experience of the world. We are usually unaware of perception and it is very fast acting. However, perception is not simply based on the input that the brain receives via the senses. Our expectations and our experience have an active influence on perception. Also, what we perceive may be changed by the context in which we see it.

Let us think about a goal-oriented activity, for example making a phone call (Figure 4.1). Upper limb muscles are activated to lift and hold the phone, while the trunk muscles stabilise the body, and the larynx produces the speech sounds. At this level of the description, it is easy to forget the cognitive demands of the activity. We can only make a phone call if we can find the number, remember it long enough to dial, and if we can both produce and understand spoken words. The cognitive functions in this activity include perception, memory, motor planning and sustained attention. These all cooperate to achieve the goal. For many people with brain damage it is impairment of cognitive function, which acts as the main obstacle to using the phone.

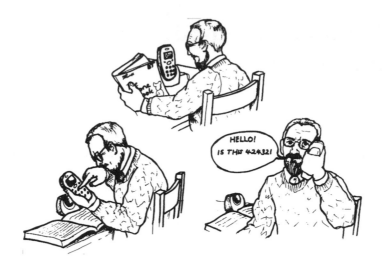

Fig. 4.1 Stages in using the telephone.

Theories of perception

Perception, together with attention, is a basic stage in cognitive processing. We must attend to the features of the environment in order to perceive or make sense of them. In cognitive psychology, there have been two main approaches to the investigation of perception: 'bottom-up' and 'top-down'.

Bottom-up theories begin with the detailed analysis of the sensory input and proceed to the integration of all this information with our stored knowledge of experience. These are known as 'data-driven' or 'stimulus-driven' theories, which consider that perception is driven by the sensory information that is available from the environment.

Early processing of the sensory input from a coffee mug, for example, is largely visual, with added tactile and proprioceptive input when we hold the mug. Auditory input is included when the mug is moved around. In the bottom-up theory, sensory processing proceeds through serial stages to higher levels where it is integrated with stored knowledge from experience. If perception depended only on bottom-up processing of all the input from the senses, the capacity of the brain would be exceeded. Also, the input from the retinal image would be too ambiguous to form the basis of our visual perception of the world around us. Bottom-up theories do not completely explain the perception of complex features of the environment such as faces.

Top-down theories of perception begin with the stored knowledge of past experience, which is compared with the incoming

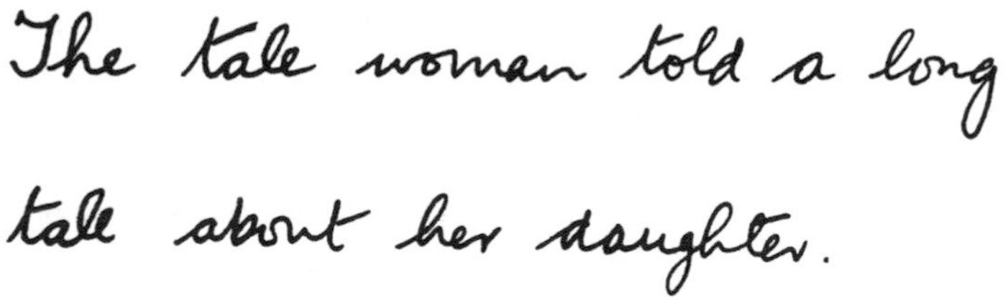

The tale woman told a long tale about her daughter.

Fig. 4.2 Top-down processing.

stimuli to the brain. Detailed analysis of all the sensory input is not required, and this means there is economy of the processing demands on the brain. These are also known as 'concept-driven' theories.

At the beginning of the twentieth century, the Gestalt group of psychologists were the first to suggest that a whole object is perceived before its parts. For example, if we see a circle with a short vertical line in the centre and short horizontal line below it, we say this is a face. At the same time, American psychologists introduced the idea that the brain is a dynamic interconnected system and each brain area can assume control for a given behaviour. It followed that the effects of brain damage depend on the extent of the damaged area rather than its location.

Support for the top-down theory of perception came later from Bartlett in the 1930s, who proposed that new perceptual input is compared with items or schemas stored in memory. An appropriate schema is then selected to match the incoming stimulus. This explains why different people perceive the same input in different ways depending on their experience. Evidence for this is the way we make sense of ambiguous information. In vision, the same input to the retina can be perceived in different ways (see Figure 4.2). In this sentence, two of the words present the same pattern to the retina, but one is perceived as 'tall' and the other as 'tale'.

In sound, the same speech output can be perceived as different. Read aloud the following two sentences:

> That noise makes me want to scream.
> Here is some vanilla ice cream.

The same sensory input can only be perceived in different ways if it is influenced by our stored knowledge, and by the context in which it is presented.

It is generally agreed that perception depends on both bottom-up and top-down processing. We interpret what the senses pick up by integration with experience. The link between perception and learned experience allows us to adapt behaviour appropriately in response to changes in the sensory input.

In people who have no sensory loss, the functional problems may originate in disordered perception or in the retrieval of stored knowledge related to the task. Normal perception is so spontaneous and automatic that it is difficult to understand the experience of impaired perception in a person with brain damage. While the effects of altered sensory input can be experienced by blindfolding our eyes or plugging our ears, understanding disordered perception is more problematic.

When the sensory input is confusing, we have to make an effort to find a solution. The responses of a group of people to looking at an ambiguous figure illustrate this (see Figure 4.3). Some may 'see' it as an old woman, and some may 'see' it as a young woman. After a time, many will 'see' it as either one or the other, or neither and say 'I will believe it when I see it'. It is these exercises that begin to make us realise what it is like for persons with perceptual problems. For them, looking at a cup and saucer may require the effort we needed to find a solution to the ambiguous figure.

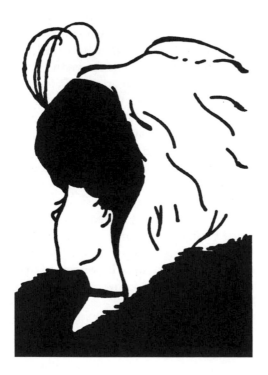

Fig. 4.3 Ambiguous figure.

Cognition in everyday function

Cognition is all the mental processes which allow us to perform meaningful activities in everyday living. A large part of our day is spent on activities that are habitual or routine. Some of these support the rhythms of daily life with established procedures while others contribute to satisfaction, for example storing our clothes in an orderly way. Non-routine habits need practice to improve until they become established. Novel situations require planning and problem solving to achieve the desired goal. The cognitive demands of routine and non-routine activities are different.

A routine task proceeds automatically with a low level of sustained attention. Most of us have a routine we follow to grab something for breakfast and prepare to leave the house in the morning. If we move house or start a new job, we then have to respond to novel situations in daily living and practice is needed to establish new routines in memory.

Non-routine tasks require an attention control mechanism with focus on a new procedure over time. If we buy a new DVD player or coffee machine, the novel procedure for their use needs extra attention demands until the routine becomes automatic. Studies of people with brain damage have shown that some may be able to perform routine activities in a familiar environment but are unable to learn new tasks. Others may be unable to organise their day because routine tasks are not triggered by the environment.

Multi-tasking requires switching of attention from one task to the other. Washing up and listening to a play on the radio are dual tasks that can be performed within the normal limits of attention. When attention capacity is exceeded, errors are made and one or more tasks break down before completion.

Cognition is involved in the planning of actions and behaviours to reach a goal at a future time. If we plan to visit a friend on her birthday, decision making (whether to go by car, or bus, or walk) and prospective memory for future actions (go on the right day) are required at the start of the journey. Finding the way involves spatial processing and memory for landmarks on the route we follow. If we choose to go by car and the route is blocked by road works on that day, additional cognitive processing is recruited to modify the plan and monitor our progress on the way until we get there.

Stored knowledge about the world is only one part of memory. Skilled actions, depending on the activation of stored procedures for their performance, are developed and improved with time and we become proficient at activities such as touch typing or playing a musical instrument. Impairment of the cognitive system affects the habits, routines and roles of people with brain damage. Cognitive impairment can have various outcomes in different individuals depending on the focal or global nature of the damage and the person's pre-morbid lifestyle.

Methods in neuropsychology

Over the last fifty years, different approaches and techniques have been used to investigate brain function. Each has made a major contribution to our understanding of the brain and of the effects of brain damage. This section will give a summary of the methods that have been developed. Examples of the use of each technique will be found in later chapters.

Models of processing in cognitive neuropsychology

One of the milestones in the study of cognition was the development of *cognitive psychology* in the 1960s. This new subject used the methods of experimental psychology to study how normal subjects take in information from the environment, make sense of it and use it (Groome, 1999). Experiments are devised to test theories and to develop models of processing in the brain, for example how we store and retrieve information. In these studies, the sensory information entering the brain from the environment under particular conditions is defined and the output response in action and behaviour is recorded. Experiments are devised to isolate the stages of processing between input and output, and test each level. In this way a model of the stages operating in one component of cognition is developed. Each stage can be considered as groups of neurones firing together, but they may or may not be located in one particular brain area.

In the 1980s, *cognitive neuropsychology* developed as a related discipline, which uses the methodology of cognitive psychology to study single persons with brain damage. The methods of cognitive neuropsychology generate flow diagrams of the stages of processing for a component of cognition, for example object recognition. The use of these models or flow diagrams is sometimes called 'boxology'.

Stages and modules

In the models developed in cognitive neuropsychology, each stage of processing is known as a module, and the flow of information from one module to the next is shown in an information processing diagram. If modules of cognitive processing are independent, it is predicted that each can be selectively impaired. For example, if a person has difficulty in recognising objects, the deficit may be at one of several different levels of processing: basic visual perception; visual structural description; semantic (meaning) representation; or lexical (name) representation (see Figure 4.4). Tests related to the individual modules in mental processing are devised in cognitive neuropsychology and these are used to identify a deficit in a particular module. For example, tests may show that basic visual perception is intact, but if the person cannot match all the forks in a drawer of mixed cutlery, this suggests impairment in forming the visual structural description of whole objects.

If a person can use objects appropriately but cannot name them, this suggests that there are independent modules for the knowledge of the names of familiar objects and for the semantic repre-

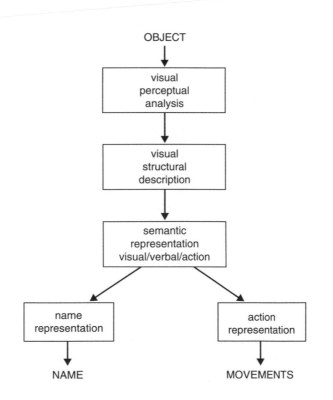

Fig. 4.4 Stages in processing, object naming and use.

sentation of the function of objects. This is known as *dissociation*. In addition, if a different person can name objects but cannot use them, this is further evidence for separate modules, known as 'double dissociation'.

The following list outlines the stages in the use of objects and the corresponding assessment.

Stage	Assessment
visual perceptual analysis	match colours, shapes, sizes
structural description	match objects
semantic representation	match objects by function
action output lexicon	demonstrate the movements for the use of an object

Cognitive neuropsychology has made a large contribution to the understanding of object recognition and language, but some areas of cognition lend themselves less well to the modular approach. When both modular and non-modular components are included in a model of processing, the modules may be coordinated by a control unit. An example of this is the model of working memory (see Chapter 8) with separate processing of visuo-spatial and of speech-based information. The control unit in this model is the central executive, which allocates attention between them. Cognitive neuropsychology is a holistic approach to brain function. There is no particular focus on the brain areas involved and the emphasis is on in-depth study of single cases.

Computer modelling in cognitive science

Cognitive science has implemented computer programs in the study of the cognitive system.

A computer program consists of a set of instructions or rules which inform the computer hardware of how to perform operations. The stages of information processing in the brain can be separated into a serial flow chart and written as a computer program. The output of the program can then be tested and compared with the response from subjects performing the same operations. In this way, models are developed which simulate cognitive processes in the brain. An example of this approach was used by Marr (1982) in the development of a theory of object recognition. Computer modelling does not mean that the brain works like a computer, but it can establish whether a theoretical process is feasible or not.

Parallel Distributed Processing, or PDP, and connectionist models are a further development of computer modelling. These models simulate the collaboration of multiple brain regions and emphasise the interconnections between them. Patterns of activity are set up within a network which then 'learns' by using rules to change the interconnections between the nodes of the network. Neural networks learn and store different patterns of processing by repeated presentation of the same input. Connectionist models can be used to predict the effect of brain damage by degrading part of the network and observing the changes in the output of the system.

A connectionist network has been compared to a collection of neurones, but the nodes of the network do not have identical properties to synapses, so the analogy can be misleading. Computer modelling supports the holistic approach to cognitive function.

Brain imaging

The structural and functional organisation of the brain can now be imaged using high resolution techniques developed over the last twenty years. These techniques are able to reconstruct two and three-dimensional spatial information about the brain. Imaging has had a major impact on research in neuropsychology.

- Computerised tomography (CT scan) uses a thin fan-shaped X-ray beam that views a 'slice' of the brain. The X-ray tube revolves round the head of the subject so that the brain is viewed from all angles. A computer combines all the views, and the changes in soft tissue at a lesion site are revealed in a single image. CT scans do not indicate functional activity in the brain but they do provide useful information about structural changes in the brain. They are now used routinely in the diagnosis of neurological disorders.

- Positron Emission Tomography (PET scan) was used extensively over the 1980s to indicate the areas where high levels of brain activity occur by sensing the local rate of blood flow. The subject receives an injection of a solution containing a positron emitting radioactive isotope which accumulates in the brain in direct proportion to the local blood flow. The results are shown on images of the brain, where brighter colours indicate higher levels of activity. The length of time available for an investigation using PET scanning is limited as the images decay rapidly with time. The subtraction method is used to identify the brain area involved in a particular cognitive function as described in the following example of imitation of movement:

Activation task A. The subject is asked to imitate specific hand movements made by the experimenter. This produces a scan of the activity of the sensorimotor and cognitive processes of interest.

Baseline task B. The subject is asked to make predetermined hand movements while watching the experimenter make the same hand movements he/she performed in task A, but this time the subject does not imitate them.
The subtracted scan, A minus B, identifies the brain area specifically associated with imitating movement.

- Magnetic Resonance Imaging (MRI) was originally used to locate soft tissue in the body more clearly than X-rays. In the early 1990s, this was developed into Functional MRI, which, like PET scanning, records the local blood flow in different areas of the brain but without the invasive introduction of a radioisotope into the body. In this technique, the increase in blood flow in an active brain area is demonstrated by the increase in the level of oxygenated blood flowing through that area. fMRI has better spatial resolution than PET scans and it can be continued over a longer period of time.

- Transcranial Magnetic Stimulation, TMS, uses a tightly wrapped, wire coil encased in an insulated sheath, which is positioned over a brain area. A large electrical current is passed through the coil, which generates a magnetic field passing through the skin and the skull to stimulate neurones in that area. The effects of TMS are brief and can only be used to explore cortical areas on the surface of the brain.

There are limitations in the use of imaging techniques. A scan may identify an active brain area during a task but the crucial operations may be the specific interactions with other brain areas. Also, the subject has to lie in a scanner, which limits the type of investigation that can be done and the time course of the investigation is short. These new imaging techniques have extended the knowledge of brain activity related to specific cognitive functions. They are useful to generate hypotheses that can be tested using other methodologies.

Stirling (2002) described neuropsychology as a broad discipline which can be divided into two approaches: clinical psychology which proceeds from damaged brain to psychological function; and cognitive neuropsychology which interprets impaired psychological function in terms of models of the stages in information processing in the brain. The methods of brain imaging, computer simulation and investigation of single case studies all contribute to extend our knowledge of the effects of brain damage on function. (A clear description of the methods of neuroscience can be found in Gazzaniga *et al.* (2002) in Chapter 4.)

Overview of brain structure and function

With the advent of brain imaging for medical diagnosis and research, knowledge of the neuroanatomy of the brain is becoming more important for communication between the occupational therapist, the neurologist and the clinical psychologist. In this section the terminology will be outlined, beginning with a brief account of the history of the naming of brain areas and their function.

The phrenologists, in the early nineteenth century, were the first to suggest that the brain was divided into 'organs' or faculties with different intellectual and emotional functions, such as cautiousness, hope, self-esteem (see Figure 4.5). Gall and his many followers believed that a highly developed faculty related to a correspondingly large area in the cerebral cortex, and this was revealed in the head as bumps in the skull overlying them. Later in the same century, the post-mortem examination of patients who had known deficits was used to name areas of the cerebral hemispheres that are concerned with the production of speech (Broca's area), and receptive aspects of speech and language (Wernicke's area). These discoveries were the first to localise language functions in the left hemisphere.

At the start of the twentieth century, neurologists described clusters of symptoms, known as syndromes, based on the detailed observation of the behaviour of people with brain damage. Frontal lobe syndrome was described by Luria, who suggested that the frontal lobes monitor and modify action and behaviour. The primary sensory and motor areas of the brain were identified by neurophysiologists in animal experiments and by neurosurgeons exploring the surface of the brain of epileptic patients to find the focus of the seizure.

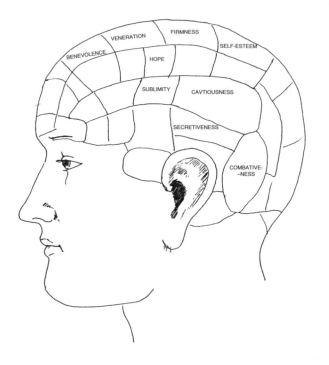

Fig. 4.5 Gall's phreno-logical map.

A detailed system for mapping the areas of the cerebral cortex was developed by Brodman in 1909. Brodman identified approximately 52 regions. These numbered areas were defined by the variation in cellular structure and connectivity in different areas of the cerebral cortex. The numbering is not systematic and probably related to the order that Brodman explored the cortex. Brodman's system of numbers is now used in neuro-imaging studies of brain function to specify location (see Figure 4.6).

Cerebral hemispheres

Anatomical descriptions divide the brain into forebrain, midbrain and hindbrain. The largest part, the forebrain or cerebrum, grows out in development to surround the midbrain and part of the hindbrain. The two halves of the cerebrum are the cerebral hemispheres, each with a surface layer of grey matter known as the cerebral cortex. Deep to the cortex, the white matter connects the neurones of the cortex with each other and with other brain areas. The two hemispheres are connected by the corpus callosum, a large body of transverse nerve fibres. This is not the only link

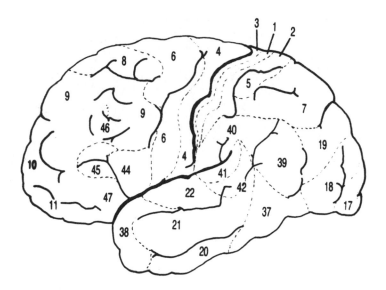

Fig. 4.6 Brodman areas.

between the two hemispheres. People whose corpus callosum was severed to alleviate intractable seizures were able to perform bilateral activities after the surgery.

Each cerebral hemisphere is divided into four lobes named after the bones of the skull which lie over them. Figure 4.7 shows the frontal, parietal, occipital and temporal lobes of the cerebral hemispheres seen in three different views.

Frontal lobe

The frontal lobe, lying in front of the central sulcus, has the major motor areas posteriorly and the pre-frontal area anteriorly:

- The motor areas include the *primary motor area*, receiving input from all the motor and sensory areas of the brain, which produces the motor commands for voluntary movement. The *pre-motor area* is important in movements that are externally generated from the changing environment. The *supplementary motor area* has a role in the initiation of movements that are internally generated. Figure 4.8a and b show the position of these motor areas in the frontal lobe.

- The *pre-frontal* area is divided into dorsolateral and ventromedial areas for the purposes of description. On the medial surface of the lobe, the pre-frontal area includes the anterior

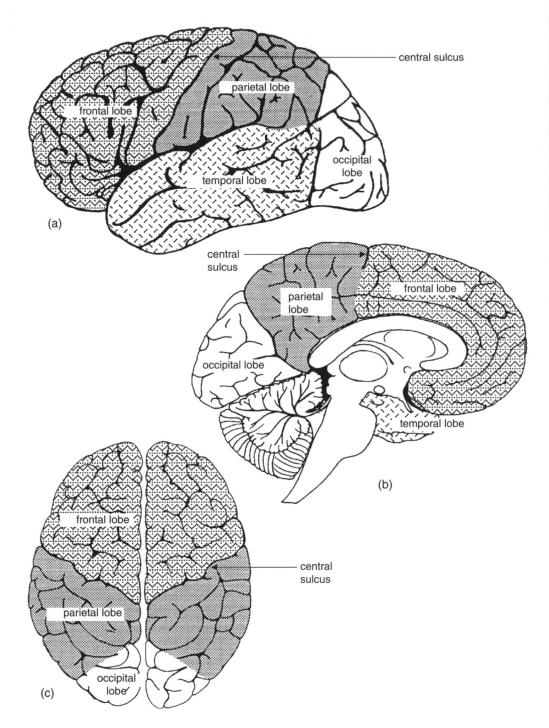

Fig. 4.7 The cerebral hemispheres as seen in three different views. a) Side view of the left hemisphere; b) Medial view of the left hemisphere seen in a section of the brain; c) Right and left hemispheres seen from above.

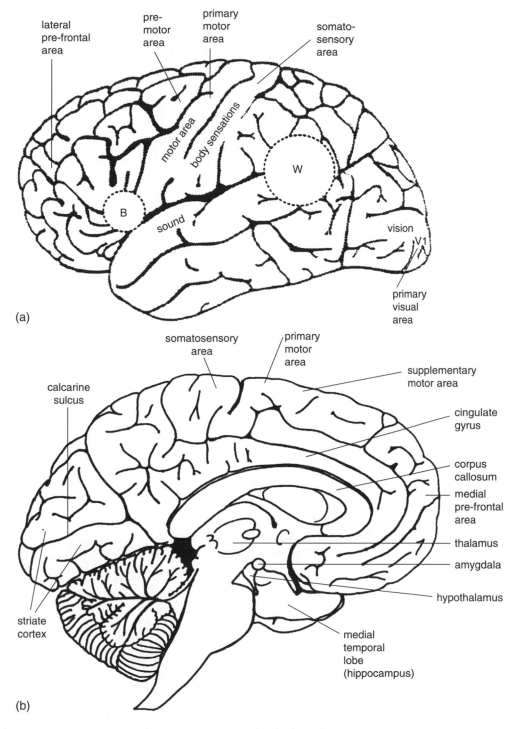

Fig. 4.8 Overview of brain areas: a) Side view of left hemisphere, B – Broca's area; W – Wernicke's area; b) Medial view seen in a sagittal section.

part of the *cingulate gyrus* (see Figure 4.8b). The pre-frontal areas are associated with the high level cognitive processes for the planning, monitoring and modifying of action and behaviour (see Chapter 10). The pre-frontal area also plays an important role in memory.

Parietal lobe

The parietal lobe lies posterior to the frontal lobe. The *somatosensory area*, immediately behind the central sulcus, receives touch, pain, temperature and proprioceptive information from all parts of the body. The output from the somatosensory area projects to the *posterior parietal cortex* for the processing of information about the position of objects in space. A pathway from the visual areas of the occipital lobe projects to the parietal lobe forming the 'where' pathway in object recognition. The parietal lobe is involved in the spatial processing of different areas of space and some aspects of short-term memory.

Occipital lobe

The *primary visual area* V1, receiving input originating in the retina of the eyes, lies at the posterior pole of the occipital lobe and extends on to the medial surface around the *calcarine sulcus* (see Figure 4.8b). This area is also known as the *striate cortex* due to its striped appearance. Surrounding the striate cortex is a large extrastriate area which analyses the colour, form, location and motion of visual information.

Temporal lobe

The *auditory cortex* A1 lies in the superior part of the temporal lobe buried within the lateral sulcus with the auditory association area surrounding it. The temporal lobe processes the visual features of objects via projections from V1 in the occipital lobe. This is known as the 'what' pathway in object recognition (see Chapter 5). Each temporal lobe contains a buried gyrus known as the *hippocampus* because it is shaped like a seahorse. The hippocampus plays an important role in memory and in the orientation of the body for route finding. The area of the parietal-temporal-occipital junction on the left side, known as 'Wernicke's area', plays a prominent role in language processing, particularly the meaningful content of speech.

Limbic system

The cingulate gyrus, amygdala, anterior thalamus, hypothalamus and hippocampus are all parts of the complex limbic system which can be seen on the medial aspect of the cerebrum and in sagittal sections of the brain. The *cingulate gyrus* arches over the *corpus callosum*, which is a mass of nerve fibres linking the right and left hemispheres (see Figure 4.8b). This area, together with the pre-frontal cortex, plays an important role in the executive functions for the planning and monitoring of action and behaviour. The *amygdala* processes emotional stimuli independently and also interacts with other brain areas to produce emotional responses.

Right/left differences in processing

The dominant hemisphere, usually the left, tends to be larger and heavier than the non-dominant hemisphere. The inputs to the two sides from the senses and from other brain areas and the spinal cord are largely the same, so any difference between the two must lie in their capacity to process different types of information.

The dominant *left hemisphere*, in most people, is dominant for all language functions: reading, writing, the understanding and the production of speech. These functions involve the processing of sequences, letter by letter, word by word and so on. The left hemisphere is also associated with the processing of sequences of action, which are the basis of most of our functional move-ments. For example, in the activity of pouring water from a jug, the actions of reach, grasp, lift, pour, lower and release are per-formed in series. The sequential processing involved in language, numeracy and movement means that the left hemisphere has been called the 'analyser'.

The non-dominant *right hemisphere* has a greater capacity to process visual and spatial information that cannot be described in words. The recognition of objects, the position of body parts during movement, and the spatial relationships of objects and landmarks in the environment, are associated with the right hemi-sphere. The right hemisphere deals with wholes rather than parts and has been called the 'synthesiser'.

Differences in affective processing in the two hemispheres have led to the right hemisphere being called the 'emotional brain'. The right hemisphere processes the emotional information in speech and facial expression. People with right hemisphere damage may show indifference and denial of their disabilities. Those with language problems due to left hemisphere damage often show feelings of anxiety and depression, but they may be able to express and understand emotion in non-linguistic ways, for example facial expression.

The extensive interconnections between all the cortical areas mean that each lobe of the cerebral hemispheres does not function in isolation. Links occur between: sensory and motor areas of the cortex; cortical areas to sub-cortical areas, the brain stem and the spinal cord; and between right and left sides. Furthermore, each component of cognition may involve networks whose elements are located in several different cortical areas. People with disruption in the same brain location can have different outcomes, depending on the extent of cerebral damage, and on the other brain areas that are involved.

Note on terminology

The terms hemiplegia and hemiparesis are associated with motor and sensory loss as a result of cerebral lesions on one side of the brain. In the organisation of the central nervous system most of the tracts of nerve fibres between the brain and the spinal cord cross to the opposite side. This means that lesions of the right hemisphere lead to left hemiplegia, and left hemisphere lesions lead to right hemiplegia. In the accounts of brain damage in this book, the location of the lesion will be described rather than the side of hemiplegia. It must be emphasised that cognitive deficits resulting from brain damage may occur with or without motor and/or sensory loss.

The cognitive system

The complex cognitive system functions as a whole, with subsystems interacting at different levels of processing. In order to gain an understanding of cognition, the system can be broken down into components. Each underlying cognitive skill supports effective function, and impairment in one subsystem impacts on the system as a whole.

The occupational therapy frameworks for practice classify the client factors that may affect performance in areas of occupation. In the OTPF framework, the global and specific mental functions are summarised as follows:

Global mental functions	Specific mental functions
arousal, orientation, personality, drive, motivation	attention, memory, perception, recognition, concept formation, motor planning, psychomotor responses, emotions, body image, self-esteem, language, calculation functions

This book considers arousal and the specific mental functions drawing on research studies in these areas in neuropsychology. The acquisition of the language skills and calculation functions will not be included. Cooperation with the speech and language therapists is imperative when there is impairment of language skills and memory.

Research topics in neuropsychology include perception, attention, memory, planning and problem solving. A challenge was issued by Norman (1980) to cognitive psychologists to include culture, consciousness, emotion and belief systems in research in cognition. Since that time, emotion has become a research topic in cognitive science (Gazzaniga *et al.*, 2002, Chapter 13) and the way that attention can operate at both conscious and unconscious levels is an emergent area of research.

The organisation of the chapters in this book is designed to reflect the cognitive abilities that are the concern of occupational therapy practice. The components of cognition will be grouped under the following headings:

- Visual perception: object and face recognition
- Spatial abilities: constructional skills, body scheme, topographical orientation
- Attention: sustained, selective and divided attention
- Memory: working memory, long-term memory, everyday memory
- Purposeful movement: models of praxis, motor planning, intention
- Executive functions: routine and non-routine action and behaviour, self awareness

Each of the Chapters 5 to 10 will cover normal cognitive function in one of these areas, together with the related disorders and their effects on function. At the end of each chapter, suggestions for assessment and intervention will be outlined.

Summary

1. Cognition is all the mental processes concerned with the acquisition and use of knowledge. New information entering the brain is organised and classified. Knowledge is stored and retrieved at a later time. Cognitive processes allow us to interact with each other and with the changing environment, to make decisions, and to perform meaningful actions and behaviour.

2. In cognitive psychology, theories and models of the stages of the flow of information in the brain have been developed. Cognitive neuropsychology has extended these models based on the study of single cases of people with brain damage. Another approach to the study of cognition uses computer programs which simulate parallel distributed processing.

3. Knowledge of the anatomy of the brain and the associated terminology form a useful basis for the study of cognition and facilitates communication between the members of the multi-disciplinary team. The use of CT, PET and fMRI brain imaging techniques for diagnosis and research has allocated function to specific brain areas during the operation of cognitive functions. However, it must be remembered that two people with damage in the same area of the brain can have different outcomes depending on the size of the lesion and the interaction with other areas.

4. The complex cognitive system can be divided into components for purposes of understanding and to allow the occupational therapist to develop appropriate intervention strategies. Future research will tell us more about the way the cognitive components interact.

5 Visual Perception, Recognition and Agnosia

Visual perception gives meaning to all the information entering the eyes. Vision plays a major role in the total perception of the environment and the brain has a larger area of cerebral cortex devoted to the processing of vision than any of the other senses. In the constantly changing visual environment, we perceive individual objects, people and landmarks as the same, whatever their position, illumination or distance from us.

The adaptability of visual perception was dramatically illustrated in an experiment when subjects wore spectacles with inverting lenses. After several days, the subjects had adapted to the upside-down view of the world. They were able to move around normally and perform all daily living activities. Our ability to instantly recognise the features of the visual environment seems to be so easy that it is difficult to appreciate how many complex processes are involved. To represent a scene in drawing or painting we have to think about size, depth, distance, light and shade (see Figure 5.1). The great landscape painters in the early nineteenth century were the pioneers for the representation of these features on a flat canvas. The impressionist painters were able to create three dimensional scenes using flat planes of colour.

Looking around a room, each object is isolated from its background and from other objects adjacent to it. As we look out of the window, we can decide where a house ends and a tree begins, if they are overlapping. When we move about, landmarks are recognised and obstructions are avoided. The recognition of objects is associated with meaning and function for their use. In social interaction we recognise faces and associate them with the names of the people we know. Complex cognitive processing is involved to convert the retinal image into our perception of the three-dimensional world.

The person with visual perceptual deficits functions below the expected level but is often unaware of any problem. When objects are only partially exposed to view, or are seen from unusual angles, there is difficulty in recognising them. Poor object recognition leads to problems with daily living tasks, particularly when

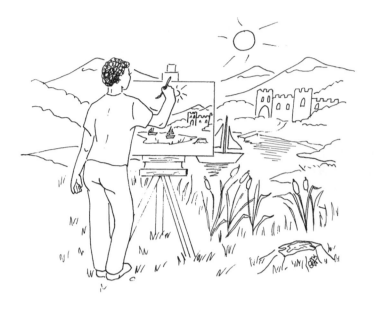

Fig. 5.1 Painting a scene.

several objects are used. In some cases it is possible to recognise objects from touch or from a verbal description. Face recognition problems affect the ability to communicate with others, leading to isolation and loss of independence. The basic visual functions of visual acuity and coordination of eye movements, as well as a deficit in visual perception, may be an underlying factor in the impairment of any component of cognition.

Early visual processing

The retina of each eye receives a two-dimensional image of the visual field ahead. The role of visual perception is to convert this constantly changing image into a three-dimensional object or scene which has meaning. The features that form the perceptual analysis of the environment are colour, shape, size, depth, figure ground and motion. Early screening for shape and colour can be done with a form board (see Figure 5.2). The brain-damaged person is asked to fit coloured wooden shapes of different form into corresponding shapes on the board.

Sensory information about the surface texture and the direction of lines and edges also contributes to visual perception. Outlines of landmarks are isolated from their background. Perceptions of objects are stable even when they are seen in different views.

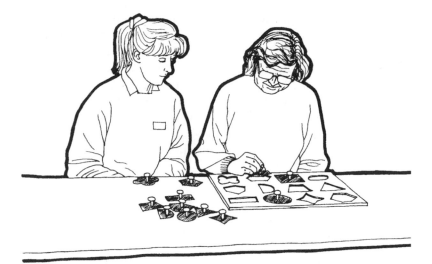

Fig. 5.2 Assessment of shape using a form board.

Colour

Colour in the visual environment gives added meaning. Colour perception is different from colour blindness, which is a retinal defect. In child development, the toddler learns that the colour and the form of particular objects are associated with their function. Even in different lighting conditions, familiar objects do not change their colour. Similar items that can be present in different colours, for example coins or food in jars, depend on colour discrimination for identification. When there is loss of colour perception, the world is seen as shades of grey, and vision is reported as 'not clear' even though visual acuity is normal. Loss of colour can occur in one half of the visual field. A photograph of a bunch of flowers is then seen with one half in colour and the other half in white.

Selective impairment of colour and shape has been described in some people with cerebral damage. This suggests that in early visual processing, colour is processed separately from shape. The inability to recognise colour, in the absence of retinal defects, is known as *achromatopsia*, or colour agnosia. The person with colour agnosia is unable to match colours, or sort different shades of the same colour. In severe form, which occurs in bilateral posterior lesions, the visual environment is seen as black, white or grey. Some loss of colour discrimination, particularly in the blue end of the spectrum, is common in cerebral lesions. An apparent loss of colour perception in the right hemiplegic person is more likely to be due to a colour-naming problem. If colour perception is impaired, faces and common objects can usually be recognised from other features, but problems arise in the use of money when bronze and silver coins appear the same. In sorting out clothes, the person relies on tactile cues and cannot colour match or coordinate separate items. There is difficulty in distinguishing foods in jars and in the selection of items, such as tins of soup or beans, from a shelf in the supermarket. Mistakes are often only realised from the smell and taste of food when the tin is opened.

Figure ground

In the 1920s, the Gestalt psychologists first proposed that perception is organised to produce 'good form'. They introduced the term 'figure ground'. In the visual world, we perceive whole objects set in a background. All the items and objects we use must be isolated from the surfaces they are on and from other objects that overlap them. The three mugs shown in Figure 5.3 are the 'figure', and the tray is the 'ground'.

Visual perception segments the environment into what is figure and what is ground. It is the grouping together of the elements of colour, form and depth that produces the figure and separates it from the ground. Many visual illusions are pictures where the figure and the ground can be exchanged. Figure 5.4 can be perceived as a vase or two faces in silhouette, depending on whether the black area or the white area is coded in the brain as the ground, respectively. A person with impairment of figure ground has difficulty in picking out objects when they are surrounded by others, for example a fork in a drawer of cutlery. The person cannot find

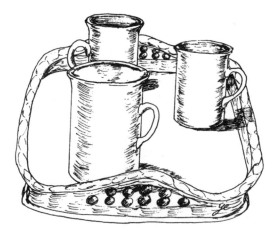

Fig. 5.3 Perception of depth and figure ground.

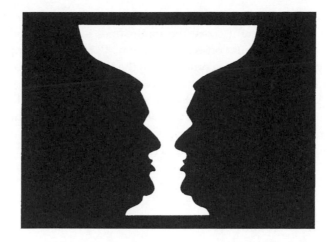

Fig. 5.4 Figure ground, two different interpretations.

things, for example the soap in the bathroom, a comb in a drawer or a cup in a cupboard. In dressing, items of clothing cannot be isolated from the bedcover they are lying on, especially a white T-shirt lying on a white sheet.

Activity

Look around the room you are in and count the number of objects that you can see. Then count how many of the objects are over-lapped by other objects. Move to the other side of the room, where you see different views of the same objects and at different distances. Note the shadows cast by the light from the window or lamp falling on the objects, and how the textures of surfaces change in the distance. All these features contribute to visual perception of the environment.

Depth perception

Depth perception comes partly from the difference in the image of an object received by the brain from the retina of each eye. There are, however, other clues in the visual field which provide information about depth. If one object partly obscures another, the complete object is perceived to be nearer. When similar objects appear to be different sizes, the larger ones are perceived to be nearer, and the smaller ones further away. Parallel lines appear to converge and textures become finer in the distance. The mugs on a tray in Figure 5.3 illustrate these clues to depth perception.

The perception of depth is basic to constructional ability and finding our way around (see Chapter 6). Movement in the environment gives clues about depth. When sitting in a moving car, nearby features of the visual scene, such as telegraph poles, appear to move by quickly, while distant trees appear to move slowly.

Perceptual constancy

Perceptual constancy is the feature of visual perception that allows us to recognise shapes and objects as the same when presented in a variety of conditions. Size discrimination is part of form constancy. We can distinguish the same shape seen in different sizes from other shapes or objects. My table appears the same size when I stand one metre away, or six metres across the room. As I move about the room, I do not see the table moving about, even though the image of the table on my retina is changing. If I tilt my head to one side, the retinal image again changes, but the table appears the same. When we view the same object in different size, orientation (see Figure 5.5) or brightness, the retinal image is different but we recognise the object as the same. If we are shown an unfamiliar object, we can still identify it as the same object when we see it from above, from below, at an angle, and so on. This is known as perceptual constancy and without it, the visual world would be very confusing.

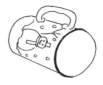

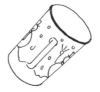

Perceptual constancy may be explained by the additional information provided in the background context. Optical illusions occur when the context triggers inaccurate perceptual constancy. People with deficits in form constancy have difficulty in recognising familiar items or objects when they appear in unusual orientation and without a background. There may be problems in kitchen tasks in selecting the appropriate item and using it correctly. In dressing, a garment may not be recognised if it is upside down or inside out.

Motion

Visual perception includes the interpretation of movement occurring in the environment. Movement separates items from their

Fig. 5.5 Object constancy.

background. It may be easier to recognise a person in a crowd if he or she is moving. We observe wind direction from the moving trees. The direction of movement of a bus is known from the sequence of images projected onto the retina. We can estimate the speed of traffic from the movement of vehicles along the road. This perceptual processing of motion is an important part of our total visual perception.

Case study (Zihl *et al.*, 1983)

A case was reported of a woman who had selective impairment of motion perception. MP had brain damage revealed in a CT scan as bilateral lesions in the temporal lobe and parieto-temporal junction. She was able to match for colour and shape, and had normal tactile and auditory perception but she experienced selective loss of motion perception, particularly stimuli moving at high speeds. Movement was perceived as a series of static snapshots with moving objects appearing in one position and then another. The tea she poured into a cup appeared to her like a glacier and she failed to notice when it was overflowing. Unable to cross the road safely, she became confined to her home and was misdiagnosed as agoraphobic.

No similar severe cases have been reported but it has been shown that transcranial magnetic stimulation (TMS) over the visual cortex can affect the ability to judge whether a stimulus moves to the left or right. This condition of *akinetopsia* may only occur in bilateral lesions. Case studies of the impairment of colour perception without loss of motion perception have been reported. Therefore, the case study described above supports a double dissociation and evidence for separable processing of colour and motion.

In summary, the perception of colour, shape, figure ground, depth, motion and perceptual constancy form the early bottom-up processing which interacts with top-down processing from the environment for recognition.

Visual object recognition

Recognition of an object depends on the formation of a mental representation that is:

- Three dimensional
- Independent of size, orientation, brightness or distance from the viewer
- Sensitive to movement in different directions
- Accessible to stored representations of the object in memory

The access to stored representations of all the objects we have encountered can be compared with the recognition of a bar code at the supermarket checkout. However, this system would put an impossible overload on the storage of 'templates' in memory. The categorisation of items and storage of a central description of an object that represents a category, known as a prototype, leads to a more economical approach.

Top-down approaches in object recognition have emphasised the importance of contextual information. Textures, surfaces and lines in the visual environment give meaning to what we see, and these are interpreted in the context of the changing scene around us. Gibson (1979) proposed that surfaces and objects 'afford' action. The affordance of an object is what it offers as a possibility for action. A handle affords grasping, the shape of a jug affords tipping (see Figure 5.6). Some people who have poor semantic knowledge of the meaning of objects can use them by activating the action system by a direct route from perception to action (Riddoch & Humphreys, 1987). The importance of contextual information means that functional assessments in occupational therapy are facilitated in the person's home environment using objects known to him or her. Performance is also affected by the number of objects present, the spatial arrangement of the objects, the complexity of the task and the environment (Toglia, 1989).

Studies of object recognition have used: laboratory experiments involving visual search and feature analysis; computer programs with algorithms, which operate on two-dimensional images to reach a three-dimensional representation; and the assessment of patients with visual recognition problems to identify the stages

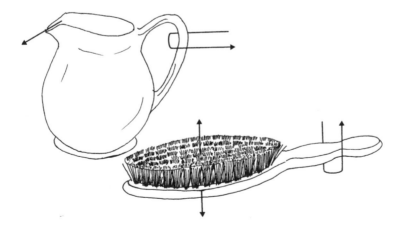

Fig. 5.6 Affordance of a jug and a brush.

in processing. The cognitive neuropsychology approach has produced an information-processing model of object recognition (Ellis & Young, 1988) which forms a useful basis for the assessment of object recognition problems in occupational therapy (see Figure 5.7).

- Viewer centred representation is the output of early visual perceptual processing. This representation is determined by the observer's viewpoint and this level is intact if the person can copy line drawings and match objects.
- Object centred representation is the mental processing of objects that can be recognised in any view. This representation

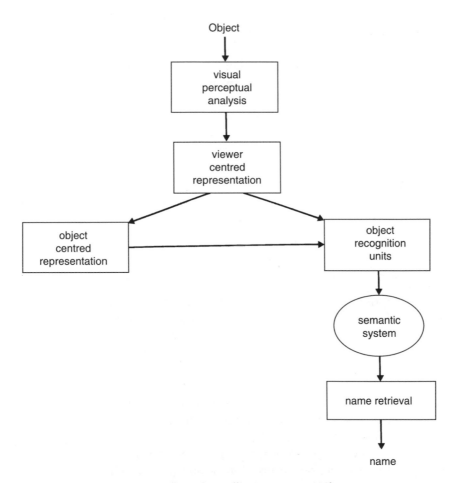

Fig. 5.7 Model of object recognition (based on Ellis & Young, 1988).

is independent of specific viewpoint. The level can be assessed by matching and recognition of the same object in different views.

- Object recognition units are stored descriptions of known objects in memory. The outputs from the viewer centred and the object centred representations are compared with these stored descriptions for recognition of a known object.
- The semantic system is the processing of stored knowledge of the meaning and function of objects. The semantic representation may also be accessed from tactile input or from a verbal description of an object. If there is no deficit in the semantic system, objects can be matched by function, and can be used appropriately.
- Name retrieval is achieved by access to the lexicon of the names of known objects. Interruption at this level means that an object may be recognised and used, but cannot be named.

There is considerable evidence for the separation of structural, semantic and naming levels of processing in object recognition, with some cross modular processing (known as cascade). Problems in the use of objects can arise due to impairment at any of these three levels. Naming problems demand cooperation with a speech and language therapist. A person with a naming problem may be able to recognise objects by touch and he or she can mime their use. This is known as *optic aphasia*.

In Chapter 9, we will consider the output from semantics to the action system which activates the movements associated with the use of objects.

What and where pathways

Early visual perceptual processing occurs in the occipital lobe. In the 1980s, two independent projections were identified extending from the occipital lobe to the temporal and to the parietal lobe. Studies in neuropsychology have focused on the differences in processing in the two pathways:

- The ventral pathway extending to the temporal lobe relates to the perceptual processing of objects for recognition, known as the 'what' stream.
- The dorsal pathway to the posterior parietal lobe relates to the perceptual processing of the position of objects in space, known as the 'where' stream.

Case study (Goodale & Milner, 1992)

DF, aged 35 years, had bilateral lesions in the occipital lobes as a result of the inhalation of carbon monoxide from a leaky gas heater. She was unable to recognise objects, drawings or pictures. She was able to name an object when it was put in her hands, so it was not a naming problem. Also, she had no loss of visual acuity. DF was assessed on her ability to perceive the orientation of a three-dimensional object. In this experiment she was asked to view a circular wooden block with a slot cut in it. The orientation of the slot could be varied (see Figure 5.8 below).

In the first condition, DF was given a card and asked to orient her hand so that the card fitted the slot, for example hold the card horizontal if the slot was horizontal. She was unable to do this, orienting her hand vertically for a horizontal slot (see Figure 5.8a.).

In the second condition, DF was asked to insert the card into the slot. She was able to do this accurately, orienting her hand correctly before contact with the slot (see Figure 5.8b).

Goodale & Milner concluded that we use two different sources of perceptual information, one to identify objects and the other to localise objects in space for guiding action. DF was able to respond to the visual processing that guided movement but impaired in the route to the temporal lobe for object recognition. This case study provides evidence for the dissociation of object perception and object action.

(a)

(b)

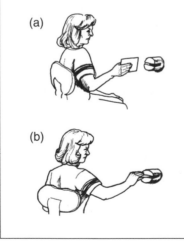

Fig. 5.8 Dissociation of recognition and action: a) Unable to match the orientation of the card and the slot; b) Correct orientation for action.

More recent studies have shown that the guiding of action is limited to the uni-axial slot and does not apply when the action involves a shape with two axes. The difference between processing in the what and where pathways has been modified to include interaction between them and the inclusion of other modules.

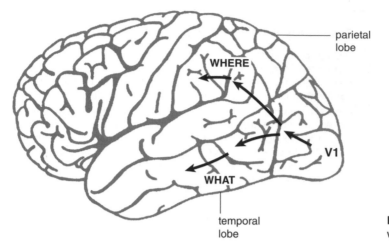

parietal
lobe

WHERE

V1

WHAT

temporal
lobe

Fig. 5.9 What and
where pathways.

Some authors have also suggested that the dorsal pathway should be called the 'how' stream, describing its role in mediating action. When the dorsal stream is impaired in people with parietal lesions, they can recognise objects via the ventral stream but cannot use visual information to guide action for their use. This is known as *optic ataxia*. Figure 5.9 shows the what and where pathways extending from area V1 in the occipital lobe.

Visual agnosia

Visual agnosia is the inability to recognise familiar objects by sight in the absence of any significant visual or intellectual impairment. Agnosia means literally 'no knowledge'. Pure agnosia is clinically rare but many single cases of visual object agnosia have been reported in cognitive neuropsychology.

Visual object agnosia was first divided into two main types by Lissauer in 1900. The two types are:

- *Apperceptive agnosia* is a failure to form a stable perceptual representation of objects. Recognition problems are based on impairment of visual perception. Patients cannot match or copy shapes or objects. They are able to identify and name objects from touch and sound.
- *Associative* (semantic) *agnosia* is the inability to recognise familiar objects when visual perception is intact. Patients are able to copy and draw shapes and objects. They can name objects from verbal descriptions of their structure, but cannot describe

the function of objects. A mental representation can be formed but it cannot be associated with stored knowledge of objects and their use.

Apperceptive agnosia usually occurs in right hemisphere lesion and associative agnosia with left hemisphere lesion, particularly the left temporal lobe. Associative agnosia may be explained as a disruption of the 'what' pathway.

In the 1980s more complex tests for visual agnosia were developed, for example presentation of objects in unusual views, with minimal features, in silhouette and superimposed shapes. Tests of object function have included matching a test item (rolled umbrella) with an object with the same function (open umbrella) or a visually similar object with a different function (walking stick). These studies have identified variations of the types of visual object agnosia within the two main divisions.

Case study (Humphreys & Riddoch, 1987)

HJA had bilateral occipital lesions as a result of a stroke following an appendicectomy. He could move around without bumping into objects and could reach out to pick things up but he was unable to recognise familiar objects from vision. He was able to identify objects by touch and to give detailed definitions of named objects. He could copy drawings, taking hours to draw them and producing considerable detail. His perception of the fine detail was intact but he was unable to relate them to the whole object for recognition. When he made an accurate copy of a line drawing of an owl, he said that he saw a complex pattern of lines and he could not identify the owl.

Based on the comprehensive study of HJA, Humphreys & Riddoch proposed that in normal object recognition the global form of an object is coded first and then the local fine detail is integrated into the form for recognition, introducing the term *integrative agnosia*.

An account of object agnosia developed by Farah (1991) focused on whole or part-based processing for recognition. Farah suggested that object recognition, which involves both whole and part-based processing, lies in the middle of the continuum between face recognition (whole-based processing) and the recognition of words (part-based processing). This hypothesis is based on a review of all published cases in the literature. People with object agnosia often have either face agnosia or alexia in addition, but these other two conditions usually occur alone.

Some people with visual agnosia are able to recognise some objects better than others. Farah and other authors have reported individuals with agnosia who could name drawings of living things but could not name non-living items. These studies, supported by PET scan studies, have suggested that different processes or parts of the brain are involved in the recognition of living compared with non-living things. This observation is known as a category specific impairment. So far, there has been no report of a double dissociation, that is, a person who can recognise non-living but cannot name living things. More recent research has pointed to the use of line drawings for stimuli in these tests as the source of the apparent category specificity. Living things are items that are more familiar as words than images, and drawings of them are more complex than those of non-living things.

It is difficult to imagine the problems confronting people with agnosia who are surrounded by a very confused visual environment. For some, nothing seems familiar and basic forms blend into confusion. For others, the detail of objects obscures the outline form. This may be like looking through a telescope and trying to remember the view in different directions. Some people show a marked recovery in the first few months after onset. For others, the problem persists for the rest of their lives. Interesting accounts can be read in Humphreys & Riddoch (1987) and Sacks (1985).

The relationship between visual perceptual deficits and the performance of activities in daily living (ADL) in stroke patients has been investigated (Toglia, 1989; Edmans & Lincoln, 1990; Titus et al., 1991). The nature and the number of the perceptual tests used in each of the studies are different but the results predict that the presence of visual-perceptual deficits in right or left hemisphere lesion patients does affect ADL performance adversely.

Face recognition

The ability to recognise faces has great significance in the way we function in everyday living. Face recognition is the basis of all our interaction with other people. A face offers much more information than an object. In common with objects, a face must be processed as a visual structure and recognised as a face when seen from different views. The detail of the size, shape of the eyes, nose and mouth, and the texture of the skin, make each face unique and familiar. In a face, we are also presented with the expression of feelings and emotions, and with the movement of the lips in speech. Very early in development, a young baby makes movements of the eyes and head to follow the face of someone in his or her view and may copy their facial expressions. We can identify a family member, a friend or a colleague from the sound of his or her voice, from a fleeting glimpse in a crowd or from their unique facial expressions. The recognition of a person is supported by the integration of knowledge about the person, for example age, gender, occupation and behaviour. There are many different reasons for a failure to recognise someone but we always need to know who they are before we can remember their name.

Studies in neuropsychology have focused on the question: 'Is face recognition special and different from objects?' Some support for the distinct processing for faces is offered by studies using face inversion.

Activity

Ask a partner to lie supine on the floor and then look at the face from a position behind his or her head. Try the same situation with objects lying on a table, viewing each in normal and inverted position from the top end of the table. What difference do you notice in the view of the upside-down face compared with a reversed object?

When photographs of famous people are presented to normal subjects in normal and inverted orientation, recognition is instant for the upright position but slower when inverted. This inversion effect is much less marked with objects. The results of imaging studies on normal people have shown different areas of the temporal lobe are activated when upright faces are recognised compared with inverted ones. These observations suggest that templates in memory are stored separately for upright and inverted faces.

Early studies of the stages of processing in cognitive neuropschology, based on studies of normal people and those with problems in recognising familiar faces, led to a model of face recognition described by Bruce & Young (1986) (see Figure 5.10). More recent investigations have focused on the detail of the parallel processing of biographical information. The model shown in Figure 5.10 is based on the Bruce & Young model. The stages are:

- Visual perceptual analysis discriminates the visual elements of a face, the eyes, the nose, the mouth and so on. Disruption at

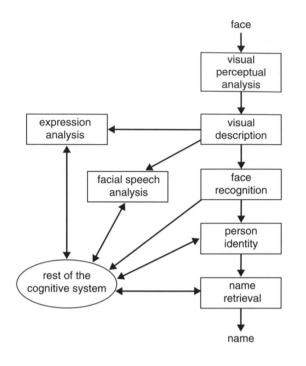

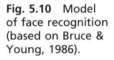

Fig. 5.10 Model of face recognition (based on Bruce & Young, 1986).

this early stage means inability to distinguish the basic features of a face, and is likely to lead to more widespread perceptual difficulties.

- Visual structural description discriminates a face as different from objects and other items, shown by the ability to match faces. Parallel processing in modules for expression analysis and facial speech movements (lip-reading) occurs at this level.
- Face recognition units contain structural information about known faces. This allows for the identification of a known face but not a particular person. *Is this a face that looks familiar?*
- The person identity nodes are stored knowledge of the identity of particular known people. *Do I know this person?* The output from the processing of facial expressions and facial speech, together with biographical information of age, culture, occupation and so on, access this level via the semantic system and memory (labelled the cognitive system).
- Name retrieval is the stage for access to stored knowledge of the names of known people. *I know this person, what is his or her name?* Disruption at this stage means the person has been identified but cannot be named.

The model shows that name generation can only be accessed from the person identity nodes, which in turn store biographical information about the person. This means that we are not able to put a name to a face without knowing other information about that person, for example occupation or relationships. This was confirmed by a study that asked people to keep a diary of problems they experienced in face recognition (Young *et al.*, 1985). The subjects never reported putting a name to a face while at the same time knowing nothing else about them. Only a few subjects could remember some information about a person but not their name.

Activity

Over a short lunch-time break in the refectory at college or work, look carefully at everyone around you. Keep a total count and note:

1. How many you can recognise
2. How many you can name
3. How many are unfamiliar

What factors determine your ability to recognise or name the members of this group?

Prosopagnosia

Prosopagnosia is the inability to recognise familiar faces in the absence of sensory impairment. In severe cases, the person cannot recognise their own family or even their own reflection. A face may be recognised as a face but not whose face it is. Sometimes, family members are not forgotten and they are recognised when the voice is heard. Loss of naming must be differentiated from pure memory loss, so that cooperation with the speech and language therapist is important.

The parallel processing of facial expressions and facial speech occurs independently from recognition based on the visual structural representation. This dissociation has been shown in people who were able to recognise the expressions of faces they could not recognise, while other prosopagnosics showed the opposite. They could not identify the expression on a face they could recognise. We need to be able to recognise a face whatever the expression at the time. There is a similar dissociation between expression analysis and lip-reading.

Another interesting line of research into face recognition is the phenomenon of covert recognition. People who are totally unable to recognise faces have demonstrated that some recognition is occurring below the level of conscious awareness. When prosopagnosic subjects were asked to learn to associate names with faces, they found it much easier to learn to associate a face with its real name than with some other name, demonstrating some unconscious recognition.

Face recognition is based on a modular system of independent processes which can be selectively impaired. PET scan studies have identified the right temporal lobe when specific faces were identified by normal subjects. Single case studies of people with prosopagnosia in the literature showed bilateral damage in the occipital and temporal lobes or unilateral damage in the same lobes on the right side.

FUNCTIONAL CONSEQUENCES

For people with visual perceptual deficits, the world is seen as unfamiliar, strange and confusing. In the home environment, activities of daily living are difficult to perform when objects cannot be recognised. The appropriate tool cannot be selected for a particular purpose. Food containers in cupboards cannot be selected by shape and colour. In dressing, items of clothing cannot be chosen, particularly when they are overlapping and lying on a bedcover. Clothes may not be recognised when they are upside down or inside out. There may be difficulty in recognising personal possessions, such as the contents of a handbag. The enjoyment of walking around the abundance of flowers in the garden is less than before.

In the outside world, items cannot be identified on the supermarket shelves and there may be difficulty in sorting the coins for payment at the checkout. In the street, the speed and distance of moving vehicles cannot be estimated accurately enough for safety. The pursuit of leisure activities may be marred by the inability to estimate the distance of the flight of a ball. Poor face recognition affects social interaction with family, friends and neighbours and leads to social isolation. Advice to relatives and friends on the importance of the voice and facial expressions can reduce the stress for the person.

Agnosia in the tactile, auditory and olfactory modalities also affects daily living. Tactile agnosia leads to difficulties when activities have to be done out of view. Doing up a back zip or finding coins in a pocket are examples of this. Work activities using equipment and machines often involve manipulative operations out of view. Auditory agnosia can lead to inability to distinguish the voices of different people. He/she may leave the vacuum cleaner or the TV on, and complain that their hearing aid is broken. Olfactory agnosia has implications for safety when the smell of gas, smoke, or burnt food is ignored.

SUGGESTIONS FOR ASSESSMENT AND INTERVENTION

Assessment

- Basic perceptual processing must be assessed prior to more complex cognitive functions. Object agnosia may manifest as inappropriate use of objects in a task, also seen in apraxia.
- Use the normal environment to screen for basic visual perceptual deficits, for example ask the person to select all the mugs of the same colour or size from a cupboard (visual scanning, colour and shape matching), or to select one specific item from a pile of clothes and identify buttons and pockets on it (figure ground).
- Observe the person whilst undertaking daily activities in the normal environment, for the functional impact of impairments in tasks such as:

  — Recognising friends and relatives by sight (prosopagnosia)
  — Locating named objects in a room (object recognition and naming)
  — Finding several of the same item placed in different orientations (object constancy)
  — Undertaking tasks using several objects (object agnosia)

- Record the type and frequency of errors in task performance, at what point a task breaks down and the context.
- Use components of standardised assessments to detect and measure specific visual perceptual deficits, and any change over time.

Assessment resources

The RPAB and the LOTCA contain tests of visual perception. Zoltan (1996) describes a series of assessments and tests for basic visual processing and visual perceptual skills. Quintana's chapter on vision and visual perception (Chapter 7) in Trombley & Radomski (2002) addresses the assessment of visual foundation skills such as visual field and oculomotor control, and basic visual perception.

Intervention

- Methods of remediation may include repeated blocked practice of exercises such as locating and naming objects, colour and shape matching, and scanning across the visual field for objects in a variety of places. Computer programs and worksheets can be used for figure ground and scanning exercises.
- There is limited evidence to support the value of programmes of remediation, in terms of the extent to which such practice carries over into functional improvement. Practice regimes may result in improvement only in highly similar tasks (near transfer) and not generalise to daily life. Grading occurs by increasing the number or variety of objects, the complexity and variety of contexts, and the reduction of cues given during tasks.
- The naming, locating and identifying of objects and people can be incorporated into daily routines, both to maximise remediation and to assist adaptation by the association of objects and people with environments.
- Adaptation to the environment and task objects, and use of compensatory techniques are important to optimise independent and safe function:

  - Providing objects and tools in specific colours to enable object recognition by association with colour (for example all mugs in bright yellow)
  - Identifying objects by touch (intact stereognosis)
  - Encouraging others to identify themselves verbally at each meeting
  - Ensuring the normal environment is uncluttered and organised consistently so that objects can be located easily

- Family involvement is very important. Participation and cooperation with adaptive measures carried over into the home can increase the individual's independence. Understanding the nature of the visual perceptual deficits will enable family members to continue to devise and refine strategies for existing and novel situations in the future.

Sources of evidence

Radomski (2002) describes interventions following traumatic brain injury, suitable for different recovery stages. Zoltan (1996)

suggests a range of intervention techniques utilising either remedial or adaptive approaches. Lee *et al.* (2001) argue the need to
incorporate both remedial and adaptive approaches and techniques to optimise functional independence.

Summary

1. Early visual processing includes colour, depth, figure ground
    and motion. There is evidence for separable perceptual process-
    ing of shape and motion. Perceptual constancy allows shapes
    and objects viewed in a variety of conditions to be perceived
    as the same.
2. Theories of visual perception have been developed to iden-
    tify processing from the analysis of the retinal image to rec-
    ognition. Other top-down processing theories emphasise the
    importance of experience. Sensory input is processed in terms
    of our expectations about the visual world.
3. The visual processing of objects follows two parallel process-
    ing streams from the occipital lobe. The 'what' stream, extend-
    ing to the posterior parietal lobe, operates on early visual
    processing for object recognition and accesses stored memo-
    ries of related objects. The 'where' stream extending to the
    temporal lobe, processes spatial information related to objects
    and mediates the guiding of action related to objects.
4. Modular models of object recognition show three main stages
    of processing in series: structural description; semantic repre-
    sentation of the meaning and function of objects; and naming.
    Each of these levels can be selectively impaired.
5. Accounts of visual object agnosia have described two main
    types: apperceptive agnosia, a failure to form a stable per-
    ceptual representation of objects; and associative agnosia, the
    inability to integrate the perceptual representation of objects
    with their function. More recent accounts of object agnosia
    emphasise the separation of global or whole-based processing
    from that related to the detail of the parts.
6. A model of face recognition describes a modular system, with
    stages from visual structural encoding to person identity and
    naming, with additional parallel modules for facial expression
    and facial speech processed via the semantic system. Person
    identity also includes knowledge of biographical information,
    for example age, gender, culture and occupation.

6 Spatial Abilities, Construction, Body Scheme and Finding the Way

Spatial ability is 'knowing where things are'. As we move around, we scan the area of space offered by the visual field of both our eyes. Once a surface or an object has been located, we analyse its relation both to our own body and to other objects around it. In the use of objects in functional activities, these spatial relations are integrated with the movements of the upper limb in reaching space. Constructional activities, when units are assembled into a two or three-dimensional whole, have a large spatial component. We may be unaware of our own spatial abilities until we try to assemble a new kitchen gadget or an item of flat pack furniture.

On a larger scale, the position of buildings and landmarks are important in finding our way around on foot, on a bicycle or in a car. The spatial relations of the features of the environment are integrated with whole body movement. We need to discriminate right and left, and mentally to be able to rotate a pathway to follow it in different directions (see Figure 6.1).

Spatial processing in everyday living has not been investigated to the same extent as other elements of perception. One reason may be the complex nature of spatial perception and the difficulty in separating the spatial element from other cognitive abilities. Attention and memory are also involved in the exploration of different areas of space. There is some evidence of separable systems for visual and spatial perception with interaction between them. The specific loss of the ability to locate seen objects is rare and it is usually accompanied by visual perceptual problems. The spatial component becomes obvious in tasks that require assembling parts together to construct a whole.

Spatial abilities demand an adequate visual field and the control of eye movements. These basic visual functions will form the introduction to this chapter, followed by consideration of the role of spatial processing in construction tasks, body movements and route finding. Unilateral neglect will be considered in Chapter 7.

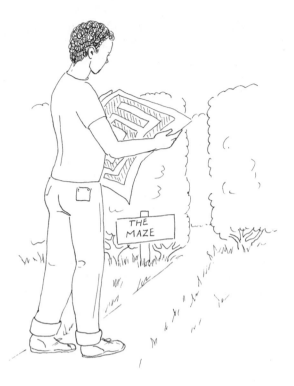

Fig. 6.1 Map of a maze.

Basic visual functions

The processing of depth, orientation and motion, described in Chapter 5, form the basis of visuo-spatial perception. These must be supported by the basic visual functions:

- Visual acuity
- Visual field
- Eye movement control

Cate & Richards (2000) emphasised the importance of these functions in a bottom-up approach for the evaluation of higher level visuo-spatial skills.

Visual acuity

Visual acuity is the ability to see small detail at all distances from the eyes. It is measured using high contrast letter charts. Acuity also depends on contrast sensitivity, which is the ability to detect the borders of objects by contrast from their backgrounds. Loss of contrast sensitivity makes reading words on a page difficult. This occurs with normal ageing and can be improved by increasing illumination.

Visual field

The visual field is the area of view of the external world seen by the two eyes without movement of the head. The visual field is like a window to the visual world. The view through the window can be scanned by movements of the eyes. Movements of the head take the window to different positions around the scene ahead and this increases the area that can be scanned. The visual field for the right and left eyes overlap in the midline, so that some light from each visual field reaches the retina of both eyes.

The visual pathway from one half of the visual field for each eye reaches the occipital lobe of the opposite side. In Figure 6.2, follow the projection from the left visual field to the inner nasal

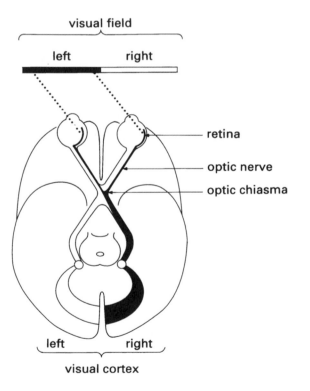

Fig. 6.2 Visual field and the visual pathway. Information from one visual field enters both eyes and projects to the visual cortex of the opposite hemisphere.

half of the left retina, and to the outer temporal half of the right retina. Now continue the same path (shown in black) onto the optic chiasma and then to the right occipital lobe. There is a mapping of the visual field in the primary visual cortex V1 around the calcarine sulcus. You should now appreciate how damage to the right primary visual cortex V1 in the occipital lobe produces 'blind areas' in the left visual field.

The following activities demonstrate:

1. How the area of the normal visual field can be estimated simply
2. The experience of the loss of a part of the visual field in both eyes

Activity

1. Stand behind a partner and ask him/her to focus on an object straight ahead. Place your fingers at different positions in the subject's visual field ahead – to either side, above and below. Ask your partner to report when the fingers are seen.
2. Cut out quarters or halves of a circle in black paper. Stick pairs of corresponding shapes onto the inner half of one lens and the outer half of the other lens of a pair of spectacles. Wear the spectacles while you walk about, write, read and make a cup of coffee. Ask someone to observe your compensatory head movements.

The loss of half the visual field, experienced in (2) is known as hemianopia. If the lesion is restricted to one bank of the calcarine sulcus in V1, there is loss of vision in one quarter of the visual field, known as quadrantanopia. Damage above the calcarine sulcus leads to a blind area in a lower quadrant, while damage below the calcarine sulcus results in a blind area in an upper quadrant of the visual field.

Small areas of cell necrosis or damage in the primary visual cortex V1 around the calcarine sulcus, produce small patches of blind areas in the visual field. These scomata often occur in traumatic brain injury. Some people with scomata are unaware of the problem if visual perception fills in the blind areas. Loss of the central area of the visual field, associated with demyelination of the optic nerve, occurs in multiple sclerosis. Diplopia (double vision) reduces the ability to discriminate form. All these changes in basic visual function affect spatial perception.

A person with a visual field defect does not see objects clearly. Many people develop strategies to overcome the partial loss of vision. Even with compensation strategies, reading often remains a problem. In scanning the page from left to right, the person with loss of the right visual field cannot make sense of the text after the first few words. The person with left visual field defect cannot start to read, or has difficulty in picking up the next line as the eyes return to the left. People with unilateral neglect have similar problems with reading but they are able to read the words when they turn their head (see Chapter 7).

Case study (Andrewes, 2001)

CG suffered a cerebral haemorrhage that resulted in quadrantanopia in the lower left half of his vision. He reported that his vision seemed fuzzy and dim in parts. When he looked ahead his vision became darker or dimmer. If he looked around, the dark left lower area interfered with the rest of his vision and everything became somehow less clear. The compensation strategy he developed was to look steadily to the left. He could not drive because cars popped up from nowhere on the left side. He was unable to see clearly enough to cut up food and could not read properly. He developed a strategy of looking steadily to the left to compensate.

Eye movements

The ability to scan the space around us depends on the control of the movements of the eyes by the oculomotor system in the brain stem, together with movements of the head. Other oculomotor functions are to: maintain binocular vision; fixate on a target ahead; follow moving targets; and maintain a stable gaze when the head moves. The extra-ocular muscles, which execute the movements of the eyes, are innervated by three cranial nerves originating in the brain stem. Projections from the occipital and frontal cortex to the nuclei of these nerves in the brain stem form a system for the control of eye movements. A stable gaze is maintained by input from the vestibular system which responds to movements of the head.

Two different types of eye movement occur in following a moving image and in scanning a static display:

- A *pursuit eye movement* is a slow movement of the eyes at the same rate as a moving image in order to keep the image on the central part of the retina. This only occurs when the eye is tracking a moving target. Pursuit movements of the eyes originate in the occipital lobes.

- *Saccadic eye movements* are made in scanning a static display. They are used to quickly direct the gaze towards an object of interest. The eyes fixate on the item, for example a group of words on a page, and then make a rapid eye movement or saccade to the next item. In scanning a larger area such as a picture, the eyes first make long saccades from the centre to the periphery, followed by shorter and shorter saccades to fixate on the detail of the picture. Saccadic movements of the eyes originate in the supplementary motor area of the frontal lobes. This area activates the brain stem nuclei of the extra-ocular muscles to produce a rapid movement of the eyes to the opposite side.

Activity

1. Ask a partner to fixate on the tip of a pencil while you move it across from left to right. Observe how the eyes move slowly as they follow the target. This is a pursuit eye movement.

2. Ask a partner to move his/her eyes in a straight line from left to right. You will see the eyes make alternating fixation and rapid saccades as they scan the path from left to right.

3. Use a small coloured ball at the end of a black wand. Ask a partner to:

   a) Follow the ball as you move it slowly in different directions – up and down, from left to right, and from right to left.
   b) Fixate on the ball held in one position.

A person with problems in scanning cannot keep their eyes on the ball.

Pursuit eye movements are used to track objects as we move them around in functional activity and to follow the course of a moving vehicle along the road. These tracking eye movements are used in sports activities and in computer games when the eyes must follow a ball or a figure as it moves towards a target. We make saccadic eye movements across the words on a page in reading. Saccades also occur when we view successive landmarks in travel on a bus or a train. The ability to maintain a stable gaze is important when the whole body moves in space. The head moves with each step in walking but the eyes keep a stable gaze ahead.

Disruption of the oculomotor system leads to slower speed of eye movements and poor visual scanning. After traumatic brain injury, the eye movements are often spontaneous and erratic. Random scanning movements lead to delay in interpreting an image. Loss of the coordination of the movements of both eyes to focus on a target may lead to double vision and poor depth perception. Poor saccadic eye movements make reading difficult.

Constructional skills

In constructional activities, single units are organised into a two or three-dimensional whole. The construction may be simply putting our clothes on in the morning. Preparing a meal has a constructional component, such as making a sandwich or laying the table. More complex constructional skill is needed to assemble a food processor, a vacuum cleaner or flat pack furniture. There are many constructional elements in maintenance and repair tasks, such as fixing a car engine or a lawn mower (see Figure 6.3).

During the assembly of units to make a whole, the location of items in the environment must be integrated with the extent and direction of the movements of the hands. The mental operations

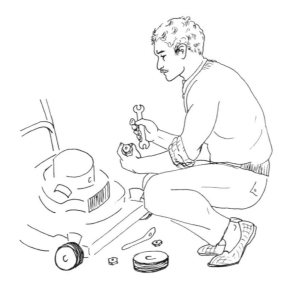

Fig. 6.3 Constructional ability.

of spatial location engage the dorsal 'where' pathway ending in the parietal lobe, described in Chapter 5. This spatial information accesses the motor areas of the frontal lobe for planning and execution of the movements. In the evaluation of constructional ability, the main difficulty is in isolating the spatial component from the motor component of the task. A further problem occurs for people with left hemisphere lesions (right hemiplegia) when the non-dominant hand may have to be used. The instructions for assembly in construction tasks need to be visual for the person with right hemiplegia, and verbal in left hemiplegia.

The investigation of constructional skills has centred around the analysis of two types of activity: drawing and building/assembly. In drawing tasks, the person is asked to copy elaborate line drawings from a model or to draw from memory. In two or three-dimensional tasks, subjects are asked to assemble coloured wooden blocks into specific designs, or build a three-dimensional construction from component blocks of different shapes and sizes. Figure 6.4 shows the assessment of constructional ability in the standardised Rivermead Perceptual Assessment Battery. The results are examined for clearly defined errors.

Errors made in two-dimensional line drawings by right compared with left brain-damaged people are as follows:

- Right brain-damaged people produce drawings that are disorganised, with distortion of the spatial relationships. Fragmented outlines are drawn with extra or repeated strokes.

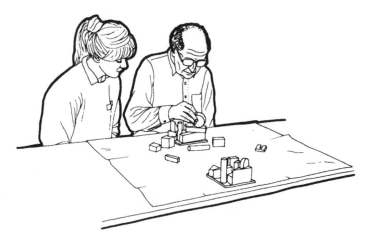

Fig. 6.4 Assessment of constructional ability. Extract (not actual size) from the RPAB by permission of NFER-NELSON (all rights reserved).

- Left brain-damaged people simplify the drawings and leave elements out. Sometimes the overall spatial layout is preserved but the drawing is lacking in detail.

A literature review of constructional performance in adults and children by Chen (1995) described significantly poorer performance in right brain-damaged adults and children compared with those with left brain damage. Performance measures included the time to completion and the number of errors of omission, addition, substitution and configuration. Attention and memory play an important role in the construction of complex drawing and assemblies. People with anterior lesions show poor planning and sequencing, which demonstrates the involvement of the executive functions in complex construction tasks.

Case study (Donnelly, 1998)

The constructional components of three functional tasks were isolated, using task analysis. The three tasks were: making a sandwich and packing a lunch box; putting on a cardigan; and setting a table. A checklist was developed of the constructional stages of each task. Thirty-five stroke patients completed the standardised visuo-spatial assessments in the RPAB, and also a functional assessment using the checklist of the constructional stages for each task. The study showed a correlation between scores on standardised visuo-spatial tests and those for the performance of the stages in the functional tasks.

Body scheme

Body scheme is the knowledge of the position of the parts of the body and the spatial relationship between them. This knowledge is based on the integration of perceptual processing of the input from vision, proprioception, tactile and pressure sensation in all the parts of the body as we move around. The discrimination of the direction of movements into upward and downward movements, right and left and so on, is part of body scheme. A standardised assessment for body scheme is found in the RPAB where the person constructs the body parts in a form board (see Figure 6.5). It is important to screen for visual perceptual deficits (see Chapter 5) and unilateral neglect (see Chapter 7) before using this test.

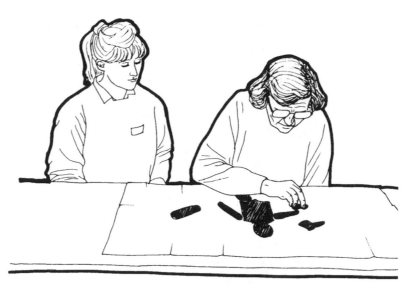

Fig. 6.5 Assessment of body scheme. Extract (not actual size) from the RPAB by permission of NFER-NELSON (all rights reserved).

The concept of body scheme has not been well defined in the literature and no unified theoretical framework for body scheme has been developed. Theories which describe the construction of body scheme have supported either a mental representation that is innate or one that is developed from sensory feedback.

The term 'body image' should be distinguished from body scheme. Body image combines body scheme with emotional and environmental inputs which produce a representation of our own body in visual imagery. This representation is often not the same as the exact physical appearance of our own body. When normal subjects are asked to draw a picture of themselves, the relative sizes of some body features may be larger or smaller than they really are. A disorder of body image has additional psychosocial and emotional factors.

Sirigu (1991) suggested that several different mental representations are incorporated into the processing of body knowledge. These are as follows:

- The lexical (name) and semantic (function) representation of each body part. *The hand is used for grasping.*
- The structural description of the position of each part in the body. *The hand is at the end of the upper limb.*
- The spatio-temporal representation of the changing positions of body parts. *The hand is moving across the body.*

Body scheme disorders

Body scheme disorder is not a single deficit and may present in different forms. The functional loss may be bilateral, or only one side of the body may be affected. Damage to the parietal lobe, the site of somatosensory integration and the termination of the 'where' pathway, has been implicated in body scheme disorder.

The classification of body scheme disorders is problematic and there is some disagreement about which disorders relate purely to body scheme without the inclusion of other perceptual deficits. Descriptions found in the literature relate to the symptoms presented rather than the specific cognitive processing that is disrupted.

- Somatognosia is a failure to recognise the parts of the body and to perceive their relative positions in space. The person with somatognosia has poor balance and equilibrium. Movements are inaccurate in the presence of normal proprioception.

- Right/left discrimination deficit is the inability to distinguish right and left in the symmetrical parts of the body. Confusion of right and left may be part of somatognosia. Many normal subjects have difficulty in right/left discrimination, particularly when asked to point to parts of body shapes presented in unconventional orientations.

- Anosognosia is the denial of the severity or even the presence of an affected limb. When asked to move the limb, the commands are often ignored, and various reasons are offered as an excuse. One subject called his arm 'George' after his son who did not work! The person is in danger of injury to the limb. Anosognosia may be part of severe unilateral neglect or body scheme disorder.

- Autopagnosia is an inability to identify the parts of the body. Finger agnosia describes when this inability is only related to the fingers. Autopagnosia may be a naming problem associated with aphasia.

In a review of body scheme disorders Corbett & Shah (1996) suggest that more definitive studies are needed of how body scheme disorders affect function. The assessments that have been developed to identify different aspects of body scheme disorder have not been validated. The incidence of body scheme disorder following CVA and its adverse effect on function makes body scheme a priority for research in occupational therapy.

Finding the way

Our ability to move from place to place in the three-dimensional world depends on a complex navigation system which operates on large-scale spatial knowledge. The orientation of the whole body in relation to the wide topographical environment which surrounds us in navigation is different from the orientation of the parts of the body in personal space (body scheme). The topographical environment is viewed from many different perspectives at different times. We must be able to navigate our way into the local supermarket whether we enter it from the pavement or from the car park.

As we explore our surroundings, working memory holds information from the environment for a few seconds at a time and retrieves spatial information from long-term memory for planning the sequence of movements along the way (see Chapter 8). Attention and visual recognition of landmarks are basic to route finding, with tactile perception offering additional information. Topographical orientation is a cognitive ability which has three stages in the acquisition of knowledge about the environment:

- Structural representation of landmarks, coded in relation to each other and to ourselves. This stage is known as egocentric or body centred. It includes the ability to judge proximity, depth and the orientation of landmarks with respect to ourselves.
- Sequencing of the landmarks in order to form a route.
- Cognitive mapping of landmarks and routes together along the way. This stage is known as allocentric or environment centred. It is independent of where we are or the orientation of the body in space. This is the basis of finding the way in real environments and of drawing a map of a route.

These three stages occur in series in child development. The young child first learns to recognise 'my house', 'my road', and 'Mary's door' at the nursery. Next he/she knows where to turn the corner on familiar routes. The third stage, which develops later, is the ability to find different paths between two places we know, or to find new routes.

We experience these stages when we move to a new home, or we arrive at college or a new place of work. We start by learning the landmarks on the way to the local supermarket, to the OT department or to the library. These short routes are then expanded and extended as we explore other parts of the area. The final stage is when we can find the way between two locations by different routes. One route is better than another when it is raining, or if you need access for a person in a wheelchair. Moving around becomes automatic.

If we get lost, we use visual or verbal strategies by looking at a map or asking the way. Some people say that they have no sense of direction, and others say that they cannot read maps. This high-lights the individual differences in the strategies we use in finding our way around. The opportunity to demonstrate this arises with first year students in their first weeks on campus, or with thera-pists at a meeting or study day held at a hospital unknown to the participants.

Activity

Form three groups of subjects. Each group is given the same task of finding the way to an unknown location and returning to the start.

Group 1 is given a simple map of the route.
Group 2 is given verbal instructions of how to get there.
Group 3 is led through the route, on the outward journey only, by someone who knows the building.

Note which group returns first (and who does not return!).
    How important was information about landmarks on the way?
    Compare the experiences of each group.

Maguire *et al.* (1997) used positron emission tomography (PET) in a study of route finding with experienced London taxi drivers. They were asked to describe the route they would drive from one named location to another around London. The results of the neuro-imaging showed a network of brain regions were active. When the active brain areas in baseline and non-topographical memory were subtracted, the hippocampus in the right temporal lobe was identified for topographical memory retrieval.

In another study using PET scans, Maguire *et al.* (1998) asked different subjects to navigate through a complex virtual reality town. After an initial period of gaining familiarity with the layout of the town, neuro-imaging was recorded during the perform-ance of various navigational tasks. When the subjects were simply asked to follow arrows through a route in the virtual town, there was greater activity in the right parietal lobe relative to the tempo-ral lobe. In another condition, when direct routes were obstructed by barriers so that detours had to be made, the left pre-frontal cortex showed activity.

The results of these imaging studies suggest that navigation is not a unitary cognitive process and it is supported by a network of brain regions, each with a specific role. Visual information from the environment reaching the occipital lobes is translated into a complex system for navigation which includes perception, attention and memory. The hippocampus in the right temporal lobe processes an environment-based representation of space which supports the ability to navigate to an unseen goal. The right parietal lobe operates on a body-centred representation to formulate correct body turns. The function of the left temporal lobe is less specified but its known role in episodic memory makes the recall of known routes most likely. The involvement of left pre-frontal cortex may be related to executive processing for planning and modifying when a direct route cannot be fol-lowed (see Chapter 10).

Topographical disorientation

Topographical disorientation is difficulty in finding the way in the large-scale spatial environment. This may be due to disturbance of one or more of the cognitive components of route finding. The origin of disorientation in the environment may be:

- *Perceptual deficit* – inability to recognise landmarks or buildings in a previously familiar environment is called topographical agnosia. Depth perception, proximity judgement and right/ left discrimination may be disrupted. Topographical disori-entation often occurs with prosopagnosia. In learning new routes, the perceptual representation of landmarks must be coded in relation to self (egocentric).
- *Memory impairment* – inability to recall landmarks and build-ings when visuo-spatial perception is intact is known as topo-graphical amnesia.
- *Spatial relations deficit* – landmarks and buildings can be rec-ognised and recalled, but there is loss of memory for their

position in space and the spatial relations between them (allo-centric). This deficit may be retrograde (relating to previously learned routes), or anterograde (relating to the learning of new routes).

Case study (Borst & Peterson, 1993)

A 67-year-old woman with a right CVA after coronary angioplasty experienced left hemiparesis and left hemianopia. Nine months after discharge from acute care, she lived at home with her husband and family. Her daughter provided much of her care, with maximum assistance in shopping and moderate assistance in bathing and dressing. She had no deficit in right/left discrimination or in the perception of depth and distance. The functional mobility of this person was restricted by extreme difficulty in finding her way around routes such as the clinic where she received outpatient rehabilitation for 12 months. She was alert, oriented and motivated to participate in treatment in occupational therapy.

Before treatment, she could follow non-spatial instructions well. Two-step directional instructions with one extra verbal prompt could be followed 50% of the time. After a four-week treatment programme her route finding ability improved using a strategy of looking at a map before starting and using directional instructions without prompting. CG achieved independence in finding her way around the clinic. Further study is needed to demonstrate carryover effects in other settings.

Visuo-spatial agnosia

Visuo-spatial agnosia occurs commonly after a stroke and has a major impact on occupational performance. For some people the problems resolve with time, while in others it persists and presents a poor prospect for rehabilitation. The definition of visuo-spatial agnosia, which covers all visual and spatial perception deficits, varies in the literature. It has been called spatial relations syndrome.

The features of visuo-spatial agnosia include difficulty in:

- Visual recognition of familiar objects and environmental landmarks
- Perception of the spatial relationships between different objects and/or landmarks
- Perception of body scheme
- Finding the way around the environment

Case study (Lampinen & Tham, 2003)

Eight individuals were studied in the period of one to six months after a right cerebrovascular accident. Visuo-spatial agnosia was identified by neuropsychological tests and by observation of difficulties in the quality of their interactions with the physical environment in everyday occupations. Each person was able to understand and answer verbal questions.

Two interviews lasting 30 to 60 minutes were conducted with each subject in one week. In the first interview, informal open-ended questions were asked about their experiences in performing everyday activities and their ways of overcoming the problems. During the second interview, the subjects were asked to choose two familiar everyday activities, for example laying the table and making a sandwich, and these were performed in the OT kitchen with video recording. When the tasks were completed, the subjects were asked to describe their experience and the difficulties they encountered. The interviews were analysed using the method of Empirical Phenomenological Perspective (Karlsson, 1993).

The participants in this study described the physical world as unfamiliar, strange and confusing. In everyday situations, which were previously taken for granted, constant effort was needed to recognise their home, family and friends. Objects were perceived as obstacles instead of tools and new ways had to be found to interact with objects. One subject could not reach objects that were close to her and felt her arms were now too short. Another person could not judge the distance from his body to a car seat so he was unable to get into a car.

The outcome of the study highlighted the importance of the development of strategies to overcome the difficulties encountered in visuo-spatial agnosia.

Unilateral neglect is another disorder related to impairment of spatial abilities. The person with unilateral neglect fails to report, respond or orient to stimuli in one side of space, usually the left. It occurs most commonly in people with lesions of the right parietal lobe. Unilateral neglect has been explained as an inability to form a mental representation of one side of space. An alternative theory describes neglect as a deficit of attention to hemispace. Spatial representation and attention theories may not be distinct since attention is required for spatial processing. The problem may also originate in failure to initiate movements to the opposite side of space. The theories of unilateral neglect will be discussed in more detail in Chapter 7.

FUNCTIONAL CONSEQUENCES

A person with a *visual field defect does* not see objects clearly. Many people develop strategies to overcome the partial loss of vision. Even with compensation strategies, reading often remains a problem. In scanning the page from left to right, the person with loss of the right visual field cannot make sense of the text after the first few words. The person with left visual field defect cannot start to read, or has difficulty in picking up the next line as the eyes return to the left.

Loss of the control of eye movements leads to slower speed of eye movements and poor visual scanning. After traumatic brain injury, the eye movements are often spontaneous and erratic. Random scanning movements lead to delay in interpreting an image. Loss of the coordination of the movements of both eyes to focus on a target may lead to double vision and poor depth perception. Poor saccadic eye movements make reading difficult.

Deficits in *constructional ability* affect all instrumental activities of daily living at some level. Meal preparation, shopping and house cleaning present problems, particularly when electrical or mechanical equipment is used. Household gadgets reduce muscular effort and joint strain but the cognitive components of the task increase when the labour saving devices have to be assembled. Dressing is a constructional task that involves holding the garments in the correct orientation to the body. Gardening has a major spatial component for handling seeds and planting an array of bedding plants. The use of cash machines demands knowledge of the layout of the key pad and the position of the slot for inserting the card. Operation of a computer requires moving the prompt around the screen to activate different icons on the desktop display and the links in a website. Many leisure pursuits, including all ball games, require the ability to track moving targets and locate the position of other members of a team.

Disorders of body scheme affect all personal care activities. Difficulty in manipulating objects in contact with the body presents difficulties in washing, toileting and dressing. Clothes may be worn inside out or back to front. Only one half of the body may be dressed. In anosognosia there is a danger of harming the body part that is ignored. People with right/left discrimination deficit have problems with using equipment that is direction oriented. In locomotion, the negotiation of stairs and kerbs is difficult without the knowledge of the distance moved by the legs at each step. This particularly affects visually impaired people since they have to rely heavily on body scheme and proprioception to estimate the depth of stairs.

Topographical disorientation produces loss of independence in daily living and also affects an individual's sense of security. Social interaction is restricted for people who cannot find their way to the shops or to join in leisure activities. The inability to manage or understand one's own environment leads to a feeling of helplessness. The loss of self-identity caused by disorientation can lead to withdrawal from human occupation. Some people do not acknowledge that they have a route-finding problem and this introduces problems of safety.

For those who experience *visuo-spatial agnosia*, the perception of the physical and social dimensions of both the person's own body and the environment are disrupted. At the person level, kerbs and stairs present a hazard for tripping and falling. Utensils are dropped off the edge of work surfaces or tables. In dressing there may be difficulty in distinguishing the top, bottom, inside and outside of clothing.

A person in a wheelchair will have problems in transferring when he or she cannot judge the distance between the wheelchair and the toilet or the bed. Wheelchair training is very difficult when the person cannot estimate distances, or turn to the right or left appropriately. The person who is ambulant may not find the way from one location to another.

SUGGESTIONS FOR ASSESSMENT AND INTERVENTION

Assessment

- Observe the individual in a variety of tasks and activities appropriate to their functional level and record the type and frequency of errors made.
- Tasks suitable to assess constructional ability include laying the table, preparing a sandwich, assembling equipment such as a food processor or vacuum cleaner.
- For body scheme disorders ask the person to point to body parts or touch one body part with another. In functional activities observe for signs that the person is ignoring body parts such as when washing and dressing.
- For topographical disorientation use familiar routes and ask the person to find their way from one point to another. Static pencil and paper tasks such as maze completion can be used but may not indicate problems when mobile in a three-dimensional environment.

- Many visual spatial tasks are complex and demand memory, attention and problem-solving skills (executive functions). These may need to be assessed.
- Standardised assessments include measures of spatial and con- structional abilities and body scheme.

Assessment resources

Standardised assessments include the RPAB, the COTNAB and the LOTCA. There is some evidence to support a correlation between scores on the RPAB and scores in the performance of stages of three functional tasks (Donnelly *et al.*, 1998). Zoltan (1996) describes a series of non-standardised functional tests for body scheme, together with comments upon their reliability and validity.

Intervention

- Visual spatial deficits frequently occur with unilateral spatial neglect and attentional problems. Intervention methods which address these impairments (see Chapter 7) may be most effec- tive in these cases.
- Training in visual scanning techniques for specific activi- ties such as reading or searching for objects can be effective (Cicerone *et al.*, 2000).
- Education of family and carers in the use of cueing (verbal and visual) and awareness of safety issues can enable successful task completion.
- Compensatory strategies include learning to check successful task completion (have I shaved both sides of my face?), using a daily checklist, or visual reminders placed in key locations. Practice and capacity for learning are important for successful use of compensatory techniques.

Sources of evidence

There is no consistent evidence that training to remediate spe- cific visuo-spatial deficits is effective. Quintana (2002) describes 'anchoring' techniques to assist with visual scanning tasks. The technique has to be learned for each specific activity and context as it does not appear to transfer or generalise. Cicerone *et al.* (2000) present a systematic literature review of cognitive reha- bilitation techniques. They make recommendations for practice standards and practice guidelines based upon the quality of evidence. Zoltan (1996) describes a range of remedial and adaptive techniques for body scheme disorders, but does not indicate their effectiveness.

Summary

1. Visual acuity, the area of the visual field and the control of eye movements are known as the basic visual functions. The ability to scan the features of the space around us demands: an adequate area of intact visual fields; pursuit and saccadic movements of the eyes; and shifts of attention.

2. Spatial processing involves the perception of depth, orientation and motion interacting with the 'where' stream for spatial location terminating in the parietal lobe. Constructional skill is the organisation of single parts to form a two or three-dimensional whole. In constructional activities, the location of objects in reaching space is integrated with spatial and temporal components of the movements of the hands.

3. Body scheme is the mental representation of the position of the parts of the body and the spatial relationship between them. Structural, semantic and lexical representations of body parts are incorporated into body scheme. The relationship between body scheme disorders and their effect on function has not been clearly defined.

4. Topographical orientation is a complex ability that involves cognitive processing at three levels: the recognition of landmarks and their spatial location; sequencing of landmarks to form mental representations of routes; and cognitive mapping of 'world centred' knowledge where landmarks and routes are combined. Neuro-imaging studies have demonstrated the role of the hippocampus in the right temporal lobe in following a route to an unseen location. Topographical disorientation, which is the inability to integrate the social and physical dimensions of the environment, leads to feelings of insecurity and withdrawal from human occupation.

5. Visuo-spatial agnosia can be defined as a global impairment of visual and spatial perception which disrupts the interaction of people with objects and with the structure of the physical environment. All everyday tasks become effortful and there is constant strife to regain the person's sense of self.

7 Attention and Unilateral Neglect

The word 'attention' is part of our everyday vocabulary. We stand to attention to be ready for action. We ask others to pay attention if there is something we want them to hear. We try to 'catch the attention' of a waiter or waitress in a restaurant. These examples illustrate how familiar we are with attention as part of our actions and behaviour. It is easy to think of attention as seeing and perceiving, but it is much more than that. Attention, acting early in cognitive processing, selects the important features in the environment and ignores all the others. The play back of an audio recording of a meeting or a social gathering includes all the background sounds we were not aware of at the time. The brain, on the other hand, selects what to listen to and what to look at from moment to moment. When there are several conversations going on at the same time, we can focus our attention on one of them. However, we may also be monitoring other conversations and react when we hear our own name mentioned (see Figure 7.1).

At times, we are distracted from the focus of attention by an unexpected stimulus such as a loud bang or a raised voice. Shifting of attention to a different location may involve moving the head and eyes or it can occur covertly without eye movement. If the telephone rings, we make a global shift of attention from the task in hand to answering the phone. Shifts of attention are important for flexibility in behaviour and action.

We perform well learnt activities on 'autopilot' with low levels of attention processing. If the same activities are performed in a noisy room or in an unfamiliar environment, higher levels of attention are required. For some, background music raises levels of attention, while for others it is a distraction.

Dividing attention between two or more tasks can be done with varying success, depending on the sensory modalities involved in each and on the limitations of the brain's attention capacity. Many people listen to the radio while driving and some keyboard operators can talk to a colleague whilst typing. There is, however, difficulty when there is a conflict in the same modality, for example

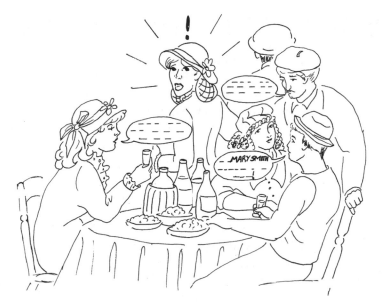

Fig. 7.1 The cocktail party phenomenon.

auditory when listening to a conversation while following a programme on television.

Attention can be internally generated and reaches consciousness when we focus on thoughts or plans. Problem solving and intellectual functions all have a large attentional component. In memory, both the registration of items and their subsequent retrieval require attention. Attention processing can be considered as a hierarchy, with each level dependent on a lower one. The basic level is arousal and vigilance, our state of readiness for action. This supports our ability to select relevant information in the environment and to shift attention from one focus to another. The highest level is the controlled processing, which sustains attention and inhibits competing response choices. In the early stages of cognitive rehabilitation, attention is a priority because deficits impact upon all cognitive functions.

Components of everyday attention

Attention is the basis of all information processing in the brain, operating on different levels. The state of arousal and alertness maintains sustained attention over long periods. Selection and shifting of attention allows us to focus our attention on matters of high priority and orient our attention to them.

Arousal and vigilance

Arousal is the physiological activity of the cerebral cortex, originating in the brain stem, when we are ready for action. The ascending reticular activating system, ARAS, is a loosely organised core of grey matter running through the brain stem with projections to all areas of the cerebral cortex via the thalamus. Sensory information is modulated by the reticular formation and the thalamus on the way to the cortex, and this determines the level of arousal. Damage to the reticular formation can result in irreversible coma.

Tonic arousal is the change in arousal level from sleep to waking, coinciding with the diurnal rhythm. The sound of an alarm clock, the sunlight appearing in the bedroom, and the movement of people, cars and trains all stimulate cortical activity and raise the level of arousal to the waking state. The reverse occurs when the stimuli in the environment decrease and we go to sleep.

Phasic arousal is a faster change in arousal, occurring in response to activity demands. The level of arousal depends on the complexity of the task and the environmental conditions. Higher levels of arousal are needed for tasks which use fine motor control or have important decision-making components. Arousal is raised if the environmental stimuli are threatening or a quick response is demanded, for example crossing a busy road. Raising arousal to very high levels for long periods leads to stress.

The relationship between arousal and performance is described as an inverted U-shaped curve (see Figure 7.2). At extremely low levels of arousal, minimal cortical activity leads to poor response to environmental change and poor motor control of action. At moderate levels of arousal, we are alert and ready for action.

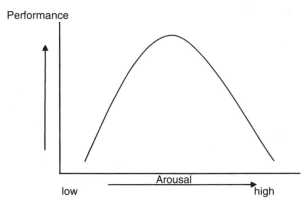

Fig. 7.2 Relationship between arousal and performance.

Beyond this optimum level, the nervous system becomes over responsive and behaviour becomes disorganised.

Vigilance is the attention that must be sustained over long periods during prolonged or repetitive activity. This sustained attention is often called 'keeping watch' and it is intrinsically linked to arousal. The maximum length of time that an individual can sustain attention is often called attention span.

The level of sustained attention varies widely, even for the same task. In motorway driving sustained attention over long periods monitors the road and detects any change that requires action. A warning of a lane closure, or the presence of a slow vehicle ahead, raises attention to the level that is required for decision making and response selection.

Selective attention

The brain is bombarded with information from all over the body and from the environment. If all of it was processed, there would soon be overload of the brain's capacity. Selective attention allows us to deal with what is important and ignore the rest. This leads to the question, 'How do we select the salient features and what happens to all the other input?' Early studies used dichotic listening and visual search to explore selective attention in sound and vision respectively.

When we are in a room full of people who are all having different conversations, we are able to attend to a conversation of interest and ignore all the other speech or music going on at the same time. This 'cocktail party phenomenon' was investigated in laboratory experiments in the 1950s, when subjects were presented with two different streams of speech, one to each ear, via headphones (Figure 7.3). The subjects were asked to attend to one channel only, right or left, and to repeat what they heard. When there were physical differences between the voices, for example the gender of the speaker or the voice intensity, the subjects were able to attend to the chosen auditory message and repeat aloud what they heard. When the two streams were in the same voice, it was difficult to separate the meaning of the two messages. These early experiments suggested that selection occurs after temporary storage and before any processing for meaning. Later experiments demonstrated some recall from the unattended channel, especially when the content was related or of high priority. When a mixture of words and numbers were presented, the recall of messages from the attended and the unattended channels was grouped for

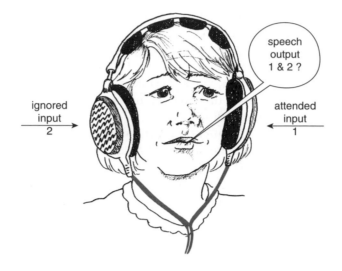

Fig. 7.3 Dichotic listening.

meaning. An alternative model was then proposed when selection occurs after semantic processing. A further development of the late selection theory was the proposition that the unattended channels are not filtered but they are attenuated, like turning down the volume on a radio or TV. The main message gets through with other information attenuated.

The level of processing of the unattended information may depend on whether it is relevant or not and on the perceptual load at the time. When the perceptual load is low, more spare attention capacity is available for semantic analysis of the unattended information before selection. Returning to the party analogy, this means our attention can be focused on the other conversations in the room when the present one becomes boring.

Activity

Put on the radio at home and read a textbook or write up lecture/case notes. Make a note of any item on the radio that catches your attention and distracts you from your work. Is it an unusual sound, a known voice on the radio, or a favourite tune? How does your experience fit into the theories of selective auditory attention?

Next, we will think about selective attention in the visual world. We spend a lot of time searching for information that is relevant to the specific task in hand. In shopping, we search for a particular

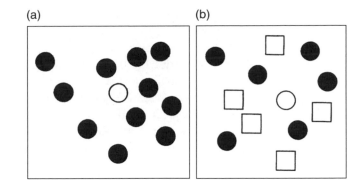

(a)   (b)

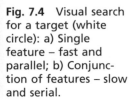

Fig. 7.4 Visual search for a target (white circle): a) Single feature – fast and parallel; b) Conjunction of features – slow and serial.

packet of cereal on a supermarket shelf; at a bus station, we search for the bus that will take us home. Selective visual attention was studied in the laboratory in the 1970s using visual search tasks. Subjects were asked to search for a target stimulus in an array of up to thirty distractors and the time to respond to the target was recorded. Both the visual features of the target, for example shape or colour, and the number of distractors were varied in different trials.

In one condition, the target and the distractors differed by a single dimension, for example a target of a white circle, together with distractors that were black circles (see Figure 7.4a). Note that the single feature difference could be in shape instead of colour. In this condition, the response time to the target was fast and it was not affected by the number of distractor stimuli there were in the display, suggesting a fast parallel selection process, called a pre-attentive mechanism.

In a second condition, the target was defined by a conjunction of features, for example colour and shape, and one of these features was shared by a variety of distractors. This is illustrated in Figure 7.4b, where the target is a white circle and the distractors are white squares and black circles. In this condition, the response time to the target stimulus was longer and it was related to the number of distractors in the array. This suggested that attention processing directed a serial search of items, one at a time, until the target was detected.

The visual search paradigm described can be compared with searching for a friend in a crowd at a railway station. A fast parallel search occurs if he or she is the only person wearing a green jacket amongst a large number of commuters in grey suits. If the crowd is more heterogeneous, additional features such as hairstyle, height and weight are used in a serial search to find the friend and this takes longer if it is a large crowd.

These experiments resulted in the Feature Integration Theory of visual attention (Treisman & Gelade, 1980) which distinguished between a fast parallel process of single features, for example colour, size orientation, followed by a slower serial process which combines the features to form objects. Visual attention provides the 'glue', which allows us to perceive an object rather than a meaningless set of features. The serial process has been described as an automatic spotlight searching an object or space. Everything within a small area of the visual field is perceived clearly compared with anything outside the beam of the spotlight. The analogy was later extended to include a zoom lens that can increase or decrease the area of the spotlight in line with task demands.

Developments of the Feature Integration Theory have suggested that selection can operate at different levels and visual search is not solely parallel or serial. Studies have shown that search can be made more efficient by ignoring stimuli that do not share the features of the target. This reflects the real world where distractors are very diverse. There is support for the view that the most important factor in visual search tasks is the discriminability between the target and the distractors. Focused attention is needed when it is difficult to discriminate between target and non-target stimuli. When the target is easy to discriminate, for example a red sports car in a multi-storey car park, a serial car-by-car search is not required to find it.

Further studies of visual and auditory selective attention have considered the role of top-down processing. Desimone & Duncan (1995) suggested that top-down processing in selective attention makes us ready to receive information that is behaviourally relevant at the expense of other input. A competition theory was proposed whereby past experience directs the detection of priority stimuli while distracting information is inhibited. An example of this is a parent who sleeps through the sound of noisy traffic in the night but always responds to the cries of the baby.

Shifting attention

The focus of our attention is constantly changing in line with the features of the environment and the task in hand. We direct our attention to different locations: to stimuli across the room or the street; to objects and people; and to our own bodies. The redirecting of attention from the current focus to another location is known as *attention shifting* or *spatial orienting*.

Shifting attention occurs in response to a peripheral stimulus, which may be a noise or the sight of a moving figure in the corner of our eyes. The unexpected sound invokes a reflex movement of the head towards the source of the noise. In vision, attention is grabbed by the moving figure and the eyes move in that direction to bring the image to a focus on the fovea of the retina. These rapid shifts of attention to a new location are automatic and they can happen with or without eye movements. Once attention has been shifted to the new location, top-down processing maintains the focus of attention there.

Object-based shifts of attention occur in task performance with multiple objects. Even the simple movement of pouring water from a kettle into a cup involves engaging attention to the kettle and then shifting attention to the cup. In some situations, covert attention shifting occurs, for example while listening to a lecture we can make way for a person who is late arriving without moving our eyes from the lecturer.

Investigations of attention shifting, in both normal subjects and in people with brain damage, described three stages: disengagement, shifting and engaging, each involving different brain areas. Apparent loss of attention shifting in people with brain damage may present as random eye movements, a fixed gaze, or inability to make voluntary eye movements, depending on the location of the damage.

Activity

This is an observation exercise of passengers on a bus or train.

Choose four of the passengers travelling with you on the way to college or work. Take a brief look at people and note the name and location of their focus of attention at that moment, for example a newspaper held in front of them. Next, record any changes in the focus of attention for each person as the journey proceeds.

What was the stimulus for each shift of attention?
What was the response?

Note any examples of dividing attention, for example changing track on an MP3 player whilst reading a book, or looking at the travel information while talking to a friend.

Could you observe any differences in the level of arousal in individuals in this group?

Compare your notes with colleagues to build up a profile of the role of attention in this example of everyday living.

Doing two things at once

Divided attention

In everyday living we are often doing more than one thing at a time. Multi-tasking is a feature of life at work and at home for many people. In this case we have to divide our attention between two or more activities that are competing. Some of us are expert at dual task performance, while others find themselves in situations where it is difficult. It may depend on what the two tasks are. Experienced drivers can successfully have a conversation with a passenger while negotiating traffic on the road. The situation is different when a driver uses a mobile phone. In a simulated study of drivers using a mobile phone, the number of errors, measured as missed red lights, was higher when talking on the phone than listening. Both talking and listening periods had more errors than listening to the radio while driving.

Case study (Spelke *et al.*, 1976)

Two students were given the difficult dual task of reading a short story for comprehension at the same time as they wrote down words dictated to them. Their progress was recorded over 17 weeks, with a total of 85 hours of practice. At first, their speed of reading was slow and their handwriting was poor. After six weeks of training for five hours a week, they were able to read with speed, handwriting improved and they showed comprehension of the text. After even more practice they were able to detect rhymes and semantically related words in the dictated lists.

Dual task experiments of this kind demonstrate remarkable ability to divide attention between two activities. The factors that have been shown to determine performance on dual tasks are task similarity, practice and task difficulty. Failure occurs when the total cognitive demands of the two tasks exceed our attention capacity. If attention processing is based on more than one resource then success or failure depends on the specific processing resources that are involved. A further explanation of success may be the formation of new strategies for performing each task to resolve the conflict between them.

Assess your own ability to do more than one thing at a time as follows:

Activity

1. Perform at the same time:

    a) A verbal and a visual task, for example recite a poem or rhyme known by heart while doing a simple jigsaw
    b) Two verbal tasks, for example listen to the radio while reading the newspaper.

    Which is easier? Why?

2. Watch your favourite soap or sitcom on the TV with a friend. At the same time, copy out your notes from a lecture or a meeting that day. At the end of the programme, relate the details of what happened in the TV programme to your friend, and ask him or her to question you on the content of the lecture.

Shared attention

Some of our work and leisure activities require sharing of attention between two or more people. Meetings at work, team games in leisure and family mealtimes, are all examples of activities where sharing of an individual's attention resources occurs in a social structure. The demands of these activities include attention shifting to each of the members of the group at different times and in different ways compared with the sustained attention when we function alone. For example, making a meal alone involves a different level of attention compared with joining a group of people to prepare a meal with family or friends. The additional visual and verbal interaction with others, combined with the demands of the practical task, has a potential effect on performance. It is important for a therapist to realise this when doing an activity with a person with brain damage. Sharing an activity is useful for the observation of an individual's level of arousal and sustained attention, but it must be appreciated that the extra attention shifting between two people increases the demands of the task.

Attention systems

Attention is part of all cognitive function. Psychologists have been considering the role of attention in cognition as far back as the end of the nineteenth century when William James distinguished between two modes of attention. The 'active' mode involves

top-down processing related to a person's goals and expectations, and the 'passive' mode is reaction to external stimuli in a
bottom-up way. Much of the research into attention since then has
studied how we identify and respond to the stimuli in the external environment. The introduction of neuro-imaging resulted in
the description of attention systems and has identified the active
brain areas.

Attention capacity

Early studies of attention processing (Kahneman, 1973) described
a capacity model with a central processor of limited capacity that
flexibly allocates attention in parallel to the activities in progress
(see Figure 7.5). The total capacity of the central processor is affected
by the level of arousal. Problems occur when the total demand of
the tasks exceeds the attention capacity. Styles (1997) compared
the capacity theory to a house with a limited gas supply. If the
rings of the gas cooker are alight when the central heating boiler
is activated, the jets on the cooker will go down. The demand of
the two appliances together decreases the amount of gas available
to the cooker. A rise in the pressure of the gas to the house would
solve the problem of the cooker, in the same way that an increase
in arousal has an effect on the total attention capacity.

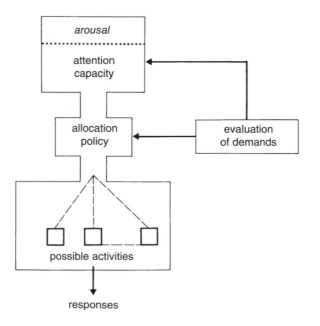

Fig. 7.5 Capacity
model of attention
(based on Kahneman,
1973).

The demands on attention capacity vary in several ways:

- *Mental effort* – novel and complex tasks demand a large share of the total attention capacity.
- *Skill* – the acquisition of skill at a task, as a result of practice, reduces the attention demands. Routine tasks that are familiar leave more capacity for an alternative activity.
- *Motivation and arousal* – increase the total capacity available for allocation. Performance increases with arousal up to an optimum.

The capacity model is a simple way of accounting for the limitations of dividing attention between two activities but it does not describe how attention is allocated by the central processor between tasks of varying difficulty. Developments of this model have replaced the single processor by multiple attention resources that are task specific. This would explain why the division of attention between two similar tasks is difficult, since they are competing for the same resource. So far it has proved difficult to isolate the stimulus characteristics of the multiple resource pools.

The capacity model does explain the effects of brain damage when overall attention capacity is often reduced. Tasks that require high mental effort become too difficult, while tasks that were well learned and familiar now become effortful. General arousal may also be reduced so that performance is slow and concentration is required in all activities. In this case, the environment needs to be controlled for the optimum performance of one task at a time.

Stimulus-driven and goal-directed attention

Since the time of Kahneman's capacity model of attention processing, most theorists have returned to the ideas of William James and divided attention into two systems. Neuro-imaging techniques have identified the different brain areas involved. Posner & Peterson (1990) described two systems: an endogenous system controlled by the person's intentions and an automatic orienting system for moving attention to priority stimuli. Posner & Peterson's description was later developed and extended by Corbetta & Shulman (2002) who described:

- A *stimulus-driven system* which detects salient stimuli in the environment and automatically shifts attention to them. This bottom-up system is activated when an important and unexpected stimulus is presented. Impairment of this system may explain why people with unilateral neglect ignore stimuli presented on the left side but they can voluntarily attend to that side.

- A *goal-directed system* controlled by the person's intentions, when the focus of attention is sustained on specific sensory information entering the brain. This top-down system is influenced by expectation, knowledge and goals. It overrides the automatic stimulus driven system in the presence of confusing or competing elements in the environment. Impairment of this system leads to distractibility.

The parietal lobe and the thalamus play a pivotal role in both systems. When an unexpected and relevant visual stimulus is presented, processing occurs in the primary visual area, V1, which projects to the parietal lobe via two routes. The direct projection in the 'where' pathway locates the position of the stimulus in the environment (see Chapter 5). The indirect route to the parietal lobe, via the colliculi in the midbrain, C, and the thalamus, Th, activates the saccadic movement of the eyes towards the location of the stimulus. When continued attentional control must be sustained, output from the frontal lobe interacts with the parietal lobe via the thalamus, and the eye movements are inhibited. This attention control by the goal-directed system is also important when organised strategies of search are required. There is some support for the view that goal-directed attention processing in the pre-frontal cortex overlaps with the central executive in working memory and the supervisory attention system in executive functions (see Chapters 8 and 10 respectively). Figure 7.6 illustrates the brain areas involved in the two systems.

Impairment of attention

Deficits in attention affect all cognitive functions. Without attention, perception is impaired and the world around us may seem confused and without meaning. Attention allows us to keep things in mind in working memory before coding in long-term memory. Recall and retrieval of items from the long-term memory store also involve attention. The close link between memory and attention means that some people who report memory problems often have an underlying attention problem. Loss of the supervisory

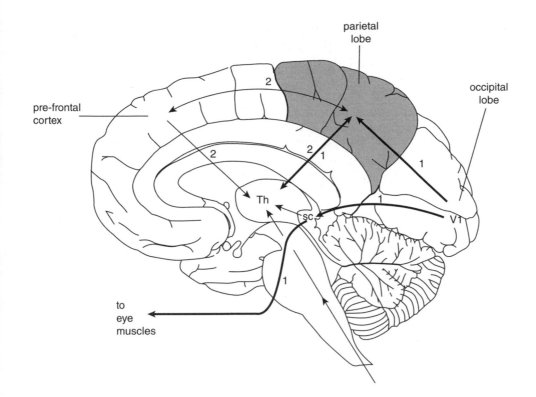

Fig. 7.6 Two attention systems. 1 stimulus driven and 2 goal directed. Th – thalamus, SC – superior colliculus.

attention control of the executive system leads to problems in decision making and flexible problem solving (see Chapter 10). This widespread interaction with all cognitive functions makes attention a priority for clinical reasoning in the rehabilitation of people with brain damage.

Reduced arousal is associated with vascular disorders, cerebral haemorrhage and tumours, which put pressure on the brain stem where the arousal system is located. Lowered arousal level is common following the resolution of coma after traumatic brain injury (TBI). High or low levels occur in changes of emotional state and motivation.

Low arousal levels lead to difficulty in the initiation of movement. Attention span is poor so that tasks do not reach termination. Sustained attention can be maintained by frequent external stimulation from the environment, for example visual or verbal cueing. Poor sustained attention means that tasks which were performed automatically over a period now require controlled effort. Only simple tasks with a clearly defined goal, reached in a short time, are possible.

People with *selective attention deficit* cannot filter out background noise and irrelevant visual stimuli. Attention is constantly drawn to irrelevant visual and auditory stimuli. Distractability is a common feature of selective attention deficit, particularly when there are a large number of competing elements in the environment. All task performance demands the shifting of attention between objects and from one region of space to another. In the absence of attention shifting, a person may maintain a fixed gaze. Even unexpected stimuli may produce no movement of the head or eyes.

In Balint syndrome, a rare neurological condition, a person loses the control of attention and orients to one object at a time. When two objects are placed in front of the person, for example a spoon and a fork, only one of them is reported, even though he or she has normal visual acuity in the entire visual field. This single report occurs both when the two objects overlap and when one is presented closer to the person than the other. Attention is drawn to one object and once engaged it cannot be moved to another one.

Case study

Rachel is a 28-year-old marketing manager who was knocked off her bicycle. She sustained facial abrasions and a fractured radius. A CT scan revealed bilateral moderate contusions in the frontal lobes. Her hospital was raising funds for an MRI scanner but there wasn't one available for a more detailed scan at that time. Whilst in hospital, Rachel read a broadsheet and a tabloid newspaper daily and used her laptop to reply to her work and personal emails. She returned to work after five weeks and started to note certain difficulties when preparing and giving presentations. She could successfully deliver a presentation that she had prepared herself and if it was based on imparting information. If her presentation was interactive or she needed to answer questions during it, she found she lost her train of thought. She also experienced significant difficulties planning joint presentations with a colleague. She was impaired in shifting and sharing attention.

FUNCTIONAL CONSEQUENCES OF ATTENTION DEFICITS

People with severe attention deficit cannot follow a daily routine without repeated external prompting. Routine tasks, which are normally performed automatically, for example brushing the hair, become effortful. The pleasure of reading a book or watching a TV drama is lost when attention cannot be sustained long enough to follow the plot. It is easier to read tabloid newspapers with features that are short. Words and images cannot be kept in mind long enough to look up the details of radio and TV programmes or telephone numbers. New memories are not encoded in recent episodic memory, so that the person cannot remember what happened earlier in that day or several days before. A conversation with one person may be enjoyed without problems, but communication may be lost when attention must be shifted and shared with a group of people talking.

Looking after young children, as either a parent or a carer, presents many problems for people with attention deficits at any level. Children's play is distracting and the continuous monitoring of young children for their safety demands both long periods of sustained attention and the ability to switch attention between the children and the task in hand.

Unilateral neglect

Neglect is defined as failure to report, respond or orient to stimuli in the space contralateral to the side of brain damage. Unilateral neglect is a complex heterogeneous disorder which occurs in varying degrees. The neglect may occur in the visual, tactile, auditory or olfactory modalities and in different spatial domains: personal, peri-personal or extra-personal space. The majority of cases are seen in right parietal lobe damage which leads to neglect of the left side of space but right side neglect has been reported. Studies in neuropsychology have been largely concerned with visual neglect.

Unilateral neglect must not be confused with a primary visual sensory deficit. The diagnosis of neglect can only be made after screening for sensory, visual field and primary motor deficits. Some people with unilateral visual neglect do have a visual field defect, which is compensated by moving the head, but others do not. Neglect is most commonly seen after a right hemisphere stroke and the estimates of the reported incidence have varied from 12% to 90% (Hartman-Maeir & Katz, 1995). In some cases the neglect resolves after a few weeks but the persistence of severe unilateral neglect is a major factor in the failure of right damaged people to respond to rehabilitation.

Pencil and paper tests for neglect include cancellation tasks. The person is asked to cross out a specific target shape, for example a large star, repeated over both sides of a page amongst distractors of different size and shape (see Figure 7.7a). People with unilateral neglect typically cancel the target shapes on the right side of the page and not on the left. In line bisection tests, the person is asked to estimate and mark the midpoint of a line drawn across a page. Neglect is shown by a deviation of the bisecting mark towards the side of the brain lesion, usually the right. When a person with neglect is asked to complete a simple form board test, only the shapes on the right side of the board will be completed. If the shapes are distributed on either side at the start, only those on the right will be attempted (see Figure 7.7b). In copying line drawings, the left side is usually omitted (see Figure 7.7c).

Extinction is a phenomenon commonly found in neglect. This can be demonstrated by asking the person to close their eyes and then touch both their hands simultaneously. Touch is then only reported on one side. When either hand is touched in isolation, the person does report it. Extinction can occur in response to visual, auditory or tactile stimuli.

Fractionation of space

Attention in the real world operates in three distinct spatial domains. These areas are described below:

- *Personal* or body space is where we use objects in contact with our own bodies, for example in toileting and dressing.
- *Peripersonal* or reaching space is the area where objects are grasped and moved around the body, for example in instrumental activities in daily living.
- *Locomotor* or far space is where the whole body moves around in the environment and when we point to or throw items. It is space related to our mobility at home, work or leisure activities. This area is sometimes known as extra-personal space.

Figure 7.8 shows the fractionation of space into these three areas. Studies of people with neglect have shown that there is a dissociation of the attention processing in each area.

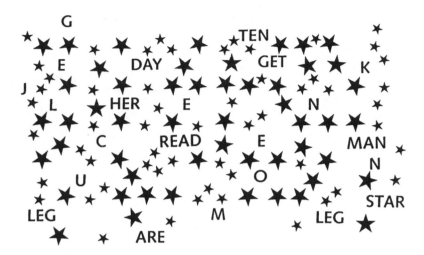

(a)

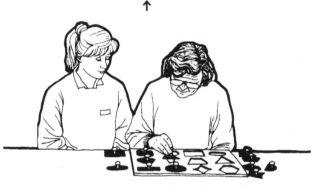

(b)

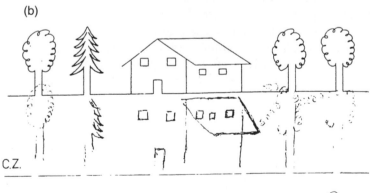

C.Z.

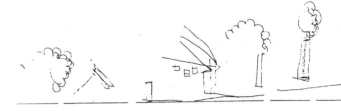

D.E.

(c)

Fig. 7.7 Tests for unilateral neglect: a) Star cancellation – extract from BIT, reproduced in reduced size by permission of Thames Valley Test Company; b) Form board; c) Copies of a line drawing (shown at the top) – reproduced from Gainotti *et al.* (1986) by permission of Oxford University Press.

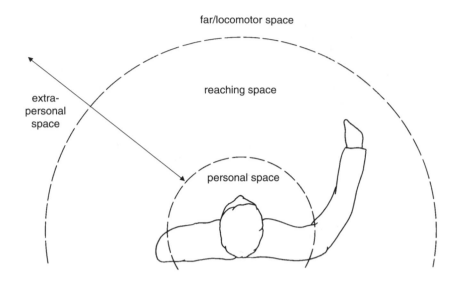

Fig. 7.8 Fractionation of space into personal, peri-personal and locomotor space.

Zoccolatti & Judica (1991) investigated the performance of twenty-six people with right brain damage on self-care activities in personal space compared with their use of objects in reaching space. The results showed that on the neglected side, the use of items in personal space, for example toileting and dressing, was less impaired than the manipulation of objects in reaching space. A single case study by the same authors showed the opposite effect, that is unilateral neglect of personal space, with unimpaired reaching space. Further, Halligan & Marshall (1991) devised a line bisection task in far space. A person with neglect in reaching space showed no problems when he was asked to bisect a line in far space using a light pointer or (as an experienced darts player) by throwing a dart. These studies suggest that unilateral neglect in the three different areas of space can be selectively impaired.

Is neglect a disorder of attention?

The person with unilateral neglect ignores one side of space (usually the left) and behaves as though it does not exist. Theories have been developed to account for this behaviour as a deficit in:

- Spatial attention
- Perceptual representation
- Pre-motor programming

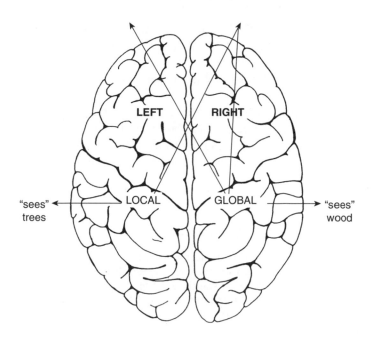

Fig. 7.9 Spatial attention, the right and left parietal lobes.

Spatial attention

In normal subjects, the right and left hemispheres each orient attention to cues in the opposite side of space with the two sides in balance (Heilman & Valenstein, 1993). The fact that neglect is more common and severe after right parietal damage suggests an additional right hemisphere dominance for attention processing which can compensate in left parietal lobe lesion (see Figure 7.9). This has been confirmed by PET scan studies, which demonstrated activity in the right parietal cortex when attention is shifted to the right and to the left, while the left parietal cortex, only, is active in shifts to the right. Further support for right brain dominance in attention was given by Heilman, who proposed that the right hemisphere is the centre for control of arousal originating in the reticular formation in the brain stem. In right brain damage, the right hemisphere is under-aroused, and this further biases attention to neglect the left side.

Differences between the right and left parietal lobes have also been shown in relation to the global and local shifts of attention. The right parietal lobe directs attention processing to the global features of items in the environment, processing groups of items simultaneously, while the left parietal lobe directs perceptual processing of the local features, item by item in a sequential way

(Robertson & Lamb, 1991). When right side damage disrupts attention to global features, the person with neglect becomes fixated on the local detail in the right hemispace and cannot disengage attention to shift to the left. This has been described as inability to see the wood for the trees.

Many of the features of unilateral neglect can be explained by a difference in attention processing between the right and left hemispheres. Studies of cueing people to the left in table-top exercises have shown benefits for people with neglect but this does not generalise to daily living.

Case study Bisiach & Luzatti (1978)

Two people with left side neglect were asked to imagine that they were in the Piazza del Duomo in Milan, which was well known to them. When they imagined standing in the square at the end facing the cathedral, they described in detail all the buildings on the right side of the square, but the buildings on the left were omitted. Next, they imagined they were standing at the opposite end of the square on the steps of the cathedral. Now they described all the buildings that they had neglected before, and omitted the buildings that were now on the left side. In each case, Bisiach and Luzatti explained this as an inability to activate the mental representations of the buildings on the left side of space and the consequent loss of visual imagery for the features on that side. Similar accounts have been described more recently by clinicians studying people with neglect. For example, a lorry driver was asked to imagine he was driving up and down the M1 motorway. When driving north, he described all the landmarks on the right side of the motorway and omitted those on the left. When driving south, he recalled all the landmarks he had previously omitted and neglected those which now appeared on the left.

These examples support the theory that in right hemisphere damage the mental representations of the left external space cannot be activated and this accounts for the features of unilateral neglect.

Perceptual representation

Our perception of the world around us depends on the formation and storage of spatial representations of external space (see Chapter 6). Also, with our eyes closed we can imagine a known external space, for example we can explore a scene we experienced on holiday. Athletes in training can use visual imagery mentally to rehearse their performance in a particular event. The formation of mental representations occurs after basic perceptual analysis and before the execution of action in that space. It has been proposed that people with neglect are unable to form the mental representation of one side of space, although not all of them show imaginal neglect as well.

In a classical study of people with neglect, Bisiach & Luzatti (1978) presented the theory that people with right hemisphere damage are unable to activate the visual and spatial representations of items present in the contralateral hemispace. This means that they may not be able to describe or think about that side of space.

Pre-motor programming

In neglect, objects placed on the neglected side are not used and movements are not made to that side. This raises the possibility that neglect originates in the loss of processing in the pre-motor areas which initiate movement towards the affected side. This impairment is called *pre-motor neglect* or hypokinesia.

Support for this theory comes from the demonstration that active movements of the limbs on the left side of the body in left hemispace can have an effect on the manifestation of neglect (Robertson & North, 1992; Robertson *et al.*, 1998; Maddicks *et al.*, 2003). The results of this limb activation therapy predict that left limb movements activate the pre-motor area of the damaged right hemisphere, which facilitates the initiation of movement to the left hemispace. An alternative explanation is that the movement of the left side limbs acts as a boost to global attention processing in the right hemisphere.

Limb activation therapy studies have used pencil and paper tests and more functional activities for the assessment of neglect. The effects of treatment have shown short-term reduction in neglect but the long-term generalisation to functional skills in daily living has not been demonstrated.

More research is needed to investigate the effect of limb movements on the remediation of neglect. Laboratory based procedures need to be modified and applied to home-based settings (Lin, 1996) bearing in mind that active left side movements are not feasible for those who also have left hemiplegia.

At the present time, there is no single theoretical account of unilateral neglect. In standard assessments of neglect it is difficult to separate attentional, perceptual and pre-motor aspects of the condition. The representational theory links neglect to loss of high-level spatial processing. Pre-motor neglect is based on a deficit in the pre-motor system for the initiation of movement to the affected hemispace. However, both spatial processing and the initiation of movement rely on the recruitment of attention to that space. The most convincing explanation is an attention deficit as either a primary or a secondary cause. A comprehensive review of the studies of unilateral neglect in neuropsychology can be found in Halligan & Marshall (1994).

FUNCTIONAL CONSEQUENCES IN UNILATERAL NEGLECT

People with unilateral neglect live and act in only one half of their surroundings. In the early stages they may have little insight into their problems and report the world as if it was complete. For some, the left half of the body feels incomplete. Spontaneous non-use movements of the left hand may occur but no functional movements are made. In dressing with sweater and trousers, only the right arm and right leg are dressed. Men with neglect shave only one side of the face and putting on make-up is a problem for women. Food preparation is difficult and only food on the right side of the plate is eaten. Reading a book is difficult when the words on the left side of the page are ignored. It may be easier to follow the information from items in a newspaper, which are presented in columns on the page.

An ambulant or wheelchair bound person may always follow a route turning to the right, and bump into things on the left. Problems occur in social interaction when any person approaching or sitting on the left is ignored. In severe cases, the progress towards independence in self-care alone is a major hurdle in rehabilitation and the prospect of return to work is poor.

Tham *et al.* (2000) interviewed four people with unilateral neglect about their experiences. They found that at any one time the people with neglect were thinking, living and acting in only one half of their life world and could not understand why they had difficulties in occupational performance. They developed feelings of alienation towards the left side of their bodies and only later began to incorporate the left arm into daily activities. Compensation strategies were most successful when they increased the understanding and awareness of the whole world around them.

SUGGESTIONS FOR ASSESSMENT AND INTERVENTION

Assessment

- Use a range of activities, some that are familiar to the person and others that are novel, as they will make different demands upon attention.
- The environment where you are conducting your assessment can be altered to facilitate attention to a task. For example, pulling the curtains around on the ward or sitting the person with their back to the window to minimise visual distractions.
- Your own behaviour may impact upon the assessment process. You may choose to advise the person that you will not talk to them whilst they are undertaking the activity to reduce distraction.

Assessment resources

Standardised assessment tools also measure different types of attention or neglect and these include the TEA, LOTCA, BIT, RPAB and the COTNAB.

Intervention

- Consider the use of cueing from the therapist and/or self-prompting to help sustain attention.
- You may choose to sit on the side that the person is neglecting to prompt and orientate.
- Repetition and practice may improve performance and increase awareness into persisting difficulties.
- There is tentative evidence to support the use of limb activation and errorless learning with neglect.

Sources of evidence

Lincoln *et al.* (2000) undertook a systematic review for the Cochrane database, exploring the evidence for cognitive rehabilitation with attention deficits following stroke. They concluded that training can improve sustained attention and alertness but did not find any evidence to demonstrate improved functional performance related to the remediation of impairments.

Maddicks *et al.* (2003) describe a single case study, which replicated previous studies of individual clients with neglect. Their findings show tentative support for the use of limb activation in the early stages of recovery, although improvements are not generalised to everyday tasks.

Wilson & Manly (2003) provide a detailed report on the use of sustained attention training and errorless learning to facilitate self-care functioning for an individual with chronic, persisting neglect. Whilst limited to a single case study, the findings of the study showed that improved functional performance was sustained after intervention. Functional performance improved despite persisting impairments.

Summary

1. Arousal is an endogenous state of preparation to act, originating in the reticular formation of the brain stem and projecting to all areas of the cerebral cortex. Vigilance is sustained attention, based on arousal, which is maintained over long periods during prolonged or repetitive activity. The frontal lobe plays an important role in the control of sustained attention.
2. Selective attention focuses on the salient stimuli in the environment whilst ignoring other sensory input. The level of processing of unattended stimuli depends on the perceptual load at the time and on their behavioural relevance.
3. Shifting attention is the ability to redirect attention from the current focus to a different object or location. Shifting attention can occur with or without eye movements and it involves three stages: disengagement, movement and engaging attention to a high priority stimulus.
4. Divided attention between two or more tasks depends on the demands each task makes on total attention resources of the brain. The outcome is affected by the modality of the sensory inputs; the nature of the response output; and the amount of practice.
5. The attention system has been divided into a stimulus-driven and a goal-oriented system, supported by different brain areas. The parietal lobe, particularly on the right, plays a central role, together with the thalamus, which filters complex sensory input for attention processing. The control of attention in the goal-oriented system operates via interaction of the pre-frontal and parietal lobes. This exerts executive control over stimulus driven action and behaviour.

6. Attention deficits affect all daily living activities. External prompting is needed for initiating, sustaining and terminating tasks. When the control of the goal-directed system is lost, people with attention deficits are distracted by irrelevant stimuli. A deficit in attention shifting may result in a fixed gaze.

7. Unilateral neglect is the inability to report, respond or orient to stimuli on one side of space, usually the left. Studies of people with unilateral neglect support an attentional deficit as the primary or secondary cause. Other explanations include an inability to activate the perceptual representations in the affected hemispace, or initiate movement to that side.

8 Memory and Amnesia

Memory is our ability to keep things in mind, and to recall them sometime in the future. We remember people's names, dates, shopping lists and the routes to familiar places. Everyday memory is also about cooking a meal in the evening, keeping track of a conversation and following the storyline of a book or a TV drama. The planning and execution of future actions and events is another important function of memory. If we plan to meet a friend at a future date, this must be remembered on the right day and at the correct time and place. We have memories of past events and experiences that we can share with others. This is important for our sense of self. Some aspects of memory are involved in almost everything we do, and the way we use it depends on our own lifestyle and experience.

Memory is often compared with systems that organise and store large amounts of information. A library of books is a static store of information that has been organised in a particular way, but retrieval is slow (see Figure 8.1). Computer systems for information storage have rapid retrieval, but they are dependent on continual update of the material if they are to remain useful. Memory is a dynamic system that is developed and modified over time, and there is no single access area in the brain.

Investigations of memory in cognitive psychology are largely laboratory based, where conditions for the presentation of the items to be remembered, and their subsequent recall, can be carefully controlled and varied in a predetermined way. The results of such rigorous explorations of memory, using lists of digits, letters, words and visual images have led to models describing the systems and processes involved in memory. In a model proposed by Tulving (1997), information is first encoded in one memory system by serial processing. For example, a telephone number may be coded as a number, linked to a person and a workspace. The number is then stored in parallel in more than one long-term memory system. Retrieval of the number occurs independently from one of these parallel systems. This is known as the serial, parallel and independent model (SPI).

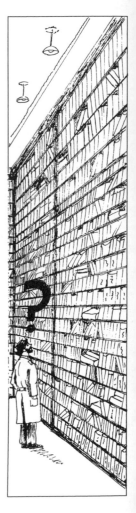

Fig. 8.1 Information storage and retrieval.

Some impairment of memory occurs in most people with brain damage. It is important to appreciate that the effects on function depend on the person's lifestyle. Also, apparent memory loss may be related to an underlying perceptual or attention problem. People with memory deficits do have residual memory skills and global amnesia is very rare. The prospect for rehabilitation largely depends on the identification of spared memory and the development of strategies to support impaired memory.

Information entering the brain from the environment is briefly registered in the sense organs as *sensory memory*, which is modality specific and it is significantly affected by sensory impairment. This processing requires attention and without it sensory memory decays. Early studies of memory proposed two types of memory store, called primary and secondary memory, which are now called short-term and long-term memory. Information from sensory memory is held for a short period in short-term memory before it is either transferred to a long-term store, or lost due to interference from new items coming in. Long-term memory retains information for periods from a few minutes to many years. Forgetting in long-term memory may be due to decay over time, or alternatively, the memory remains stored but cannot be retrieved.

Working memory

First, we will consider the evidence for a short-term memory store which is distinct from long-term memory. This will be followed by the development of short-term memory into a working memory system. Short-term memory has a limited capacity and it retains information over a period of seconds or minutes. The presence of a short-term memory store was first shown by experiments which recorded the free recall of numbers, words or pictures.

Activity

1. Make a list of 15 words, choosing concrete nouns rather than abstract words or adjectives. Alternatively, you can use 15 line drawings, for example animals, objects and tools.
    Read the list to a group of colleagues at the rate of about one word per second.
    Ask them to write down the items in the list that they can recall.

> Look in detail at the recalled words or pictures by each person in the group. Note the position in the list of each of the items recalled.
> 2. Repeat the procedure with another list of words, and this time give the group a short exercise in mental arithmetic to do before writing down the words they can recall. Again, check each of the recalled items for its position in the list.
>   Compare the results in each exercise. How successful were you with the recall of words at the beginning, middle and the end of the list? Can you explain the differences?

When this experiment was first performed in the laboratory, a plot of the percentage of items recalled against the item's position in the list showed the best recall for items at the end of the list. This is known as the *recency effect*, which was explained by the existence of a short-term memory store holding the last few items (see Figure 8.2). When the recall was delayed by the addition of a mental arithmetic task before recall, the recency effect disappeared. The additional task had produced conflict with the last few numbers. The recall of the early items in the list showed no change when recall was delayed by another task. This indicated that these items had already entered long-term memory.

A quick measure of short-term memory is the Digit Span Test. A sequence of numbers is read out at one digit per second and the subject is asked to repeat them back in the same order. The number of digits in the sequence is increased by one digit in each trial. The digit span is the largest number of digits you can get right in one

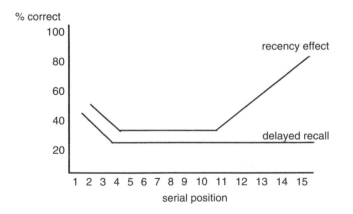

Fig. 8.2 Serial position effect in immediate (upper) and delayed (lower) recall of words.

trial. It should be noted that digit span only explores one small part of the functions of the short-term memory system.

Short-term memory was originally described as a temporary memory store of a small amount of information to hold it in mind for further analysis before entering the permanent long-term store. Studies of short-term memory in the 1970s, by Baddeley & Hitch, led to the expansion of the structure of short-term memory into a more active *working memory* system. There are two sources of information entering working memory; one is from sensory memory and the other is from long-term memory. In memory recall, information stored in long-term memory is transferred back into working memory for interpretation of the incoming information.

Working memory acts like a workbench, where verbal, visual and spatial information of both new and old memories are manipulated and integrated over a short period of time before passing on to long-term memory and to other cognitive systems. There are four main components of working memory: the phonological loop, the visuo-spatial sketchpad, the episodic buffer and the central executive (see Figure 8.3).

- The *phonological loop* stores speech-based information in a temporary store or 'inner ear'. Items are verbally rehearsed in the same order in the phonological loop before decay or passing on into long-term memory. Baddeley & Hitch found that the phonological loop was not limited by the number of items it could hold but by the length of time taken to rehearse them. This works in a similar way to a short loop of audiotape that can be replayed. In speaking and reading, several words are held long enough to make sense of the words that follow. Words can enter the phonological store directly from the ear,

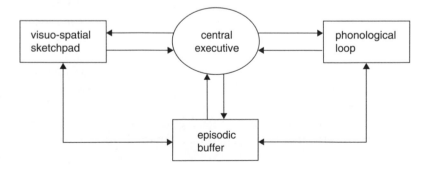

Fig. 8.3 Working memory model.

from the mental rehearsal of written or spoken words and from long-term memory.

- The *visuo-spatial sketchpad* is a temporary store of visual and spatial information entering the brain from the eye. This 'inner eye' component of working memory holds information that cannot be rehearsed verbally, such as size, shape, colour and distance, for a short time. The sketchpad is also used to inspect and manipulate visual images entering from long-term memory. If we search for lost keys, visuo-spatial images at possible locations are manipulated like 'snapshots' and compared with retrieved information from long-term memory.

- The *episodic buffer* is another component of working memory, more recently described in Baddeley (2000). The episodic buffer holds and integrates all the processing in working memory, from the phonological loop, the visuo-spatial sketchpad and from long-term memory. This component fills the gap in the general storage of visual and sound-based items into a single episode. For example, the episodic buffer integrates the visual images of people with their speech when we are watching TV.

- The *central executive* directs and controls the processing in the other components of working memory by the allocation of attention to each one. The central executive is particularly important when the cognitive demands of a task are high, or we are doing two or more things at a time.

The working memory model offers an account of how the abundance of sensory information continually entering the brain is rehearsed over a brief period of time to organise and associate it into a form that can be passed on to the other components of the cognitive system. Neuro-imaging studies have shown that the active brain areas in working memory function are widely distributed anatomically. In a PET scan study of normal subjects performing verbal tasks, the phonological store was localised in the supra-marginal gyrus of the left parietal lobe, and the articulatory loop for rehearsal in Broca's area of the frontal lobe (Paulescu *et al.*, 1993). In another study involving spatial memory, increased cerebral blood flow was recorded in the right parietal and right pre-frontal cortex (Jonides *et al.*, 1993). There is evidence to locate the central executive in the frontal lobe overlapping with the supervisory attention system (see Chapter 10 on Executive Functions).

Working memory deficits

People with working memory deficits can function in daily living when tasks do not make major cognitive demands. There is reduced capacity to process information from two or more sources simultaneously and multi-tasking is difficult. The components of working memory can be selectively impaired so that some people with brain damage may not be able to recall numbers or words that are heard, but can recall the same information when it is presented visually. Working memory can remain intact when there is severe impairment of long-term memory and vice versa.

FUNCTIONAL CONSEQUENCES OF DEFICITS IN WORKING MEMORY

Deficits in working memory affect communication. In speaking, long sentences cannot be held and rehearsed in the phonological loop long enough for understanding. The same problem affects reading. A long article in the newspaper may be difficult to understand, but comprehension is improved when it is divided into short chunks. Use of the telephone is difficult when around eleven numbers must be rehearsed before dialling. When working memory is intact, people with severely impaired long-term memory can hold a conversation and they can recall a telephone number if there is no delay after seeing or hearing them.

Problems occur at the checkout in shopping when it is difficult to inspect and choose the right coins in a purse and check the change. It may be difficult to find the way to the supermarket if visual images of landmarks cannot be integrated with retrieved long-term memory of the route. People with working memory deficit can only copy the movements of a therapist when they are done concurrently. If there is a delay before imitation, the visual and verbal input from the therapist is lost. Doing two things at a time is difficult for many people. This affects parents and carers of young children, when daily living tasks are done whilst monitoring their play. Leisure activities that involve the visual and spatial organisation of items or keeping the score may be difficult.

Long-term memory systems

Long-term memory has unlimited capacity and processes a large variety of information which is constantly updated. Items from working memory enter long-term memory where they are

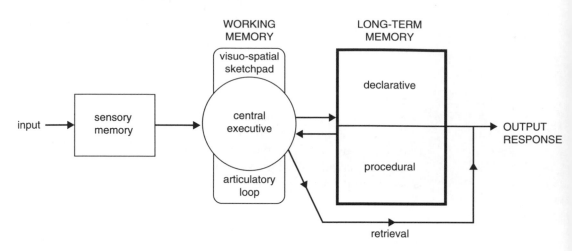

Fig. 8.4 Three memory systems.

processed for meaning and context. In reverse, stored memories in long-term memory are retrieved into working memory for manipulation and reflection before the relevant response is activated. Figure 8.4 shows how the sensory, working and long-term memory systems interact. Long-term memory has been divided into subsystems. The identification of different types of memory can assist in the prediction of functional problems and guide the choice of aids for a memory impaired person. However, the debate continues in cognitive psychology about the divisions in long-term memory and how they interact.

Procedural memory – how?

Procedural memory is the stored knowledge related to the acquisition of learned skilled activity. All the motor and language skills that we have learnt are part of procedural memory. We can speak our first language without knowing the complicated rules of grammar that are associated with it. We remember how to swim, to ride a bicycle, to drive a golf ball accurately, but we cannot explain in detail how to do it. Also, daily living involves a wide range of skills, from getting dressed, peeling vegetables to signing our name and typing, all of which are stored in memory. Procedural memory may be called 'knowing how'.

Procedural memory is *implicit*, developing through repetition and practice. It cannot be inspected consciously so it is impossible to test it by recall and recognition. Stored memories of procedures evolve into routines that are retrieved automatically in response to a specific stimulus. In the performance of motor skills, the ongoing procedure is programmed by the cortical motor areas and coordinated by the basal ganglia and cerebellum.

In most people with memory loss, procedural memory is spared. Motor skills, well learned before cerebral damage, are retained. Studies of amnesic subjects have shown that they perform badly on tests of explicit memory but they can learn new skills. This has important implications for the return to work and for the continuation of leisure pursuits in memory impaired individuals. When language skills are impaired, some people retain their first language while a more recently learnt fluent second language is lost.

The implicit nature of procedural memory is seen in people with amnesia, who show improvement in the performance of leisure tasks without awareness. When the same jigsaw is done on successive days, the level of achievement improves with repetition, even though each time the amnesic person is not aware of seeing the jigsaw before. The classic example of implicit memory in the literature is from Clarapede in 1911. He hid a pin in his hand before shaking hands with one of his amnesic subjects. She was subsequently reluctant to shake hands with him but she could not say why. This is evidence of learning without any conscious awareness of what had happened before. More research is needed into the ways in which implicit memory in people with memory deficits can be exploited in the performance of tasks.

Case study (Wilson & Wearing, 1995)

CW suffered severe memory loss following the viral infection, herpes simplex encephalitis. Brain scans showed that his left and part of his right temporal lobes had been destroyed. He had previously had a successful career as a professional musician. He developed severe amnesia for the time following the onset of his illness and was unable to acquire new memories. Also, he could not remember any episodes from his life before onset except a few facts from his childhood. He could recognise his wife but he had difficulty in recognising common objects and could not remember what had happened a few minutes before. Any conversation he had with another person was immediately forgotten. If he went out, he got lost and could not find his way back. In spite of CW's severe memory loss, his procedural memory was spared so that he could still play the piano and sightread music with great skill.

Declarative memory – what?

Declarative memory is the knowledge of people, objects, places and events. It is the memory that allows us to state whether certain facts are true or false. Declarative memory can be called 'knowing what'. It is explicit. If we are asked a concrete question, for example 'Where were you born?'" we consciously inspect declarative memory to recall the name of the place. In the laboratory, declarative memory is usually assessed by presenting subjects with test items such as words or pictures. This is followed later by free or cued recall, or recognition of re-presented test items, which may be manipulated in various ways, together with new items.

Declarative memory has been divided into two types:

- *Semantic memory* relates to knowledge of the world, without reference to how or when information was learnt. You know that Rome is the capital of Italy and bananas are yellow. Semantic memories are organised by concept and associations into a complex knowledge base and they are retrieved without context.

- *Episodic memory* relates to the memories of facts and events in their context. It refers to a particular episode or event in our lives that occurred in a particular time and place. It enables us, for example, to remember a conversation we had half an hour ago with a colleague and recall the person we met on the bus yesterday. Retrieval from episodic memory depends on the ability to recall the relevant contextual information of the time and place that it occurred, and this happens more easily in the same context that it was learnt. Riding on the same bus on another occasion may help us to retrieve knowledge of the person we met on a previous bus journey.

Some clinicians and psychologists have distinguished recent and remote episodic memory (Levy, 2001). *Recent episodic memory* is the ability to remember people, places and daily events that occurred a short time ago and they reflect a person's potential for learning new memories. A person visiting the OT department develops recent episodic memory of the layout of the rooms and the names of the staff. Recent episodic memory is the least durable of all types of memory and its impairment is often the first sign of memory loss. Older adults often experience lapses of recent episodic memory, for example they may go upstairs and then not remember why, or they may not be able to find the right spectacles to read the *TV Times*. Young people may do the same, particularly when they are stressed.

Remote episodic memory of events that occurred years before is more durable. Places and names associated with a person's family history, such as birthdays, weddings and births, from many years before, form the remote episodic memory. Memories of these events are often retained in great detail, while at the same time recent episodic memory is impaired. Some people with severe loss of cognitive function do retain remote episodic memory going back to early childhood.

Semantic and episodic interact in everyday memory. Knowledge that began as episodic becomes generalised into semantic memory over time. When you meet someone for the first time, the event is stored in episodic memory. After a time, knowledge about the person, for example colour of eyes and hair, is stored in semantic memory. This example illustrates the parallel storage of items in different memory systems. Support for the distinction between semantic and episodic memory comes from studies of people with memory loss who demonstrate impairment of episodic memory but have no difficulty in the recall of the semantic knowledge they learnt before onset. Further support comes from neuro-imaging studies which have shown that different brain areas are active during tasks involving semantic memory compared with recall from episodic memory.

Prospective memory – when?

Prospective memory is remembering what to do and when to do it. Laboratory studies have largely studied retrospective memory, but a large part of everyday memory is prospective. Stored plans for action need to be activated in the future, at the appropriate time. The time may be specific (go to a meeting at 2 o'clock), or within a period (put the plants in the garden when it stops raining). Prospective memory involves the ability to monitor time and to keep track of ongoing actions. It may also include decisions about the priority of competing plans, for example when you choose between 'have lunch' or 'complete report writing'. Prospective memory may be described as 'knowing when'.

Everyday routine tasks are mostly automatic and depend on implicit procedural memory. In non-routine activities, which have to be remembered occasionally, prospective memory is needed to activate the plan at the right time. Sometimes there is an external cue to activate the plan, for example a letterbox on the way home prompts you to post a letter. In the absence of a cue, the attention demands in working memory may affect the success or failure of prospective memory. We forget to make an important phone call on a busy day when there are many demands on our attention.

Investigations of prospective memory have included self-rating questionnaires which ask people to record when omissions occurred in their plans for the day. However, the reliability of self-rating depends on the subject's general awareness. Other studies have set subjects specific tasks, such as making a phone call at a particular time or posting a letter on a specific day, with variations in the number of actions to be remembered and in the time interval between giving the instruction and the execution of the action. There are elements of retrospective memory in the performance of future actions, for example remembering to take medication at intervals in the day is prospective, while remembering how many and the colour of each tablet is retrospective.

The success of compensatory strategies to improve prospective memory depends largely on the development of self-awareness (Fleming *et al.*, 2005). The person with memory loss needs to acknowledge the existence of problems and impaired self-awareness needs to be addressed before any external aids are introduced. Once self-awareness is established, there is motivation to use organisational devices over an extended period. Prospective memory failure is seen frequently in people recovering from traumatic brain injury.

Case study (Fleming et al., 2005)

BC, aged 19 years, developed prospective memory problems because of multiple skull fractures in a road traffic accident. He returned to live with his parents after four months of in-patient occupational therapy treatment. BC relied on family members to prompt him with daily living routines. When he left the house he forgot to take his wallet or phone with him and he forgot appointments with friends. He had several failed attempts to use a diary but later he chose an electronic organiser, including an alarm, as his compensatory tool. The alarm prompted him to refer to the organiser for details of daily chores, appointments and bill payments. The benefits of the organiser for his home and social life motivated him to continue to use it.

The long-term memory systems we have described are summarised in Figure 8.5.

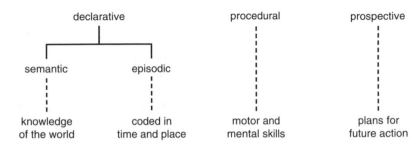

Fig. 8.5 Summary of long term memory.

Processes in memory

Memory involves three stages of processing, known as the three Rs, which operate in the long-term memory systems:

- Registration or encoding at the time of learning
- Retention or storage over time
- Retrieval and recall of information when it is required

Registration has been explored by manipulating the features and the context of the information that is learnt, and testing the subsequent recall to see what factors are most important. Information that is elaborated and processed with meaning at the time of registration increases the likelihood of later retrieval. Some of the strategies we use to improve our memory use elaboration and association, for example retracing our steps to remember where we put something, or associating the name of a person with visual imagery of his/her unique features.

Retention is a dynamic process. Stored knowledge is modified and updated by new information entering from working memory over time. Once an item has been registered in memory, subsequent forgetting could be the result of decay over time, or it could be due to interference by later learning. Recall of an event depends on the number of similar events that have occurred, rather than the time that has elapsed, suggesting that new memories interfere with interference with *knowledge of past* experience.

Retrieval involves active cognitive processing. There are two types of retrieval. Recall is a search process followed by a decision process, while recognition only involves the decision process, so that recognition is easier than recall. Retrieval is affected by the context, and items are more likely to be retrieved in the same environment as they were learnt. New learning in the hospital OT department may not generalise to the home environment.

External cueing is an important aid to retrieval of items or events from memory. Recall of the name of a person is improved if it is cued by the first letter or other information about the person. Recognition of the person from a group of names or photographs will assist successful retrieval. We are all familiar with the 'tip of the tongue phenomenon', when we know an item is in memory but we cannot retrieve it. One explanation is that the current processing does not match the stored information and fails to cue the memory. Some implicit retrieval may occur which is activated at a later time and recall is then achieved.

Levels of processing

Early studies of memory in the 1970s resulted in the levels of processing theory which proposed that the depth to which information is encoded determines what is stored in long-term memory. Information is processed at different levels ranging from shallow, for example detecting specific letters in a word, to deep semantic analysis for meaning.

In a study of the recall of words, Craik & Tulving (1975) presented a list of sixty words to three different groups of subjects.

Each group was given an additional question which oriented their perceptual processing to a particular level:

> The structural group was asked a question about the physical characteristics of the word, 'Is the word in capital letters?'

> The acoustic group was asked to process the sound of the word, 'Does the word rhyme with . . . ?'

> The semantic group was asked, 'Does the word fit into a given sentence?'

The results showed that success in retrieval of the words was greatest in the group who performed deeper semantic processing. The effect of processing depth was not only shown for verbal items but also for visual recognition. Scores were higher for face recognition when the subjects had reported the pleasantness of each face compared with reporting the structural features of each face. The levels of processing theory was originally criticised for its inadequate definition of what is meant by the depth of processing.

A later model of memory proposed parallel encoding of structural, acoustic and semantic information so that elaboration of the memory trace occurred in the three domains simultaneously. This more elaborated memory trace may create additional routes for retrieval of the item. Another explanation is that extensive input processing produces a more distinctive memory trace that is unique amongst other items in storage. It is possible that *elaboration* and *distinctiveness* operate together to facilitate retrieval in memory.

We can use different levels of processing as an internal strategy to improve our own memory. We are often confronted by a group situation with people we have not met before where we need to learn their names. Our success in remembering their names is increased if we direct our perceptual processing of each person in several ways, for example the position in the group where the person is sitting, their physical features and their behavioural characteristics. In this way we may remember the name of Peter as the one with the beard, who sits at the back of the group and asks a lot of questions. Other memory aids based on the level of processing are the use of mnemonics, association and grouping. The number of PIN numbers and passwords we have to remember is increasing, so we need to resort to these methods for making recall easier, for example by using the initials and house numbers of our friends and family.

Memory for past events is often affected by our emotional state at the time, for example the details about our first day at school. More extreme examples leave detailed memories of all the contextual features at the time. An example was hearing the news of the terrorist bombing on the London Underground in 2005. Most people in London can remember when and where they were, and who told them about the incident. Such events, known as *flashbulb memories*, may have unique registration in memory, but the frequent rehearsal and retelling of the event may account for the detail of the recall rather than a special mechanism.

Schema theory

Everyday memory involves the organisation and storage of large amounts of complex knowledge. Our success in the recall is variable. Some of our experiences are remembered, others are not, and also the recall is sometimes inaccurate or incomplete. One of the first psychologists to address the organisation of knowledge was Bartlett in the 1930s. He presented English subjects with a North American folk tale which was completely unfamiliar to Western culture. When the subjects were later asked to recall the tale, their accounts were reconstructed to make more sense in terms of their own experience. He suggested that top-down processing of the new information was incorporated into pre-stored knowledge to fit with prior expectations.

Bartlett introduced the term *schema*, which is a packet of information stored in memory representing general knowledge. Schemas are modified, updated over time and transformed into a typical form. Generalisations are made from our own experience.

Schemas can be simple or complex and they can relate to objects, situations, events or actions. A representation of simple knowledge would be a schema for the letter 'A'. A complex schema would be the knowledge related to a visit to the cinema. This complex schema may have a set of sub-schemas which include buying the ticket, finding a seat and eating popcorn. The cinema schema may be part of a larger schema for 'outings', together with a visit to the theatre or a football match. A possible schema for 'shopping' is given in Figure 8.6. The schema specifies the knowledge that is common to all shopping: place, equipment, people and actions, known as the slots. Each slot contains the concepts or actions related to it, with default values if information is not available. The optional values are acquired from particular episodes of shopping.

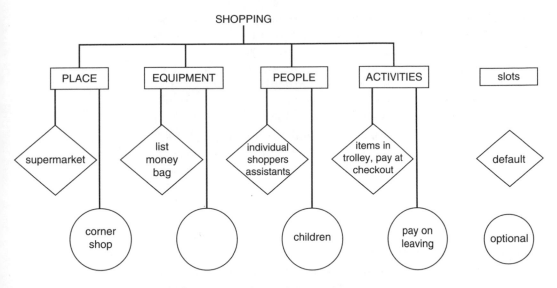

Fig. 8.6 Schema for shopping (based on Cohen *et al.*, 1993).

The way our knowledge is organised influences memory in several ways. Schemas guide the selection of what is encoded at the time of registration. Recall of the schema for a particular visit to the cinema may have ignored what you were wearing at the time, while including the knowledge of the price of the ticket. Schemas transform information from the specific to the general and this can lead to recall of the common features of an experience rather than the details of a particular episode. Top-down processing explains the errors that are made in reporting events we experience when we remember what we expected to see rather than what we actually saw.

Schema theory does account for many of the features of every-day memory and it provides a framework for the way that stored complex knowledge incorporates different types of memory. It has been criticised as being too simple and overemphasising the inaccuracy of memory. It does not explain how some complex events are recalled with great detail. The schema approach to the organisation of action sequences is discussed in Chapter 9.

Impairment of long-term memory

Memory is affected in many neurological conditions: traumatic brain injury, stroke, viral infection, degenerative disorders, cumulative brain damage in some boxers and footballers, and anoxia in cardiac surgery. Psychogenic amnesia, which occurs after ECT and in depression, will not be considered.

Visual memory is more likely to be impaired in right brain-damaged people and verbal memory in left brain damage. The relative impairment of visual and verbal memory affects both the adaptation of the person's environment and the choice of effective cues to be used by the therapist. The overall memory capacity may be reduced. One way to assess this is by reading a short story to the memory impaired person who is then asked to select picture cards which illustrate it (see Figure 8.7). This simple test can reveal the features of the person's memory function from the observation of the type and position of omissions and errors. It also gives an indication of problems with sequencing as well as total memory capacity.

Semantic and procedural memory are both durable and minimally affected by ageing. Marked changes with age may occur, however, in recent episodic memory. There is difficulty in processing newly acquired information which is not related to a person's stored semantic knowledge. This is experienced as forgetting the names of people, items of shopping and the location of objects. Older adults often report a loss of short-term memory but their problem really relates to recent episodic memory (Levy, 2001).

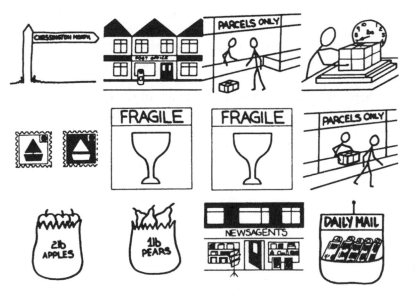

Fig. 8.7 Recall of a story in pictures – extract from COTNAB reproduced in reduced size with permission of Nottingham Rehab.

Amnesia

Amnesia is the term used to describe a severe impairment of long-term memory in the presence of relatively preserved cognitive abilities. The term *anterograde* amnesia (AA) refers to the impairment of memory for events and experiences since the onset. *Retrograde* amnesia (RA) refers to loss of memory for the period before the onset. This distinction into two types gives the means to decide whether the problem is related to learning new material or to inability to retrieve past information. If the amnesia is a learning disorder, the person will have AA but no RA. If the cause of amnesia is a retrieval deficit, the memory loss will be both anterograde and retrograde. In reality, amnesics vary a great deal in the relative severity of anterograde and retrograde loss.

There is some evidence that the underlying causes of amnesia are linked to damage in two different areas of the brain (see Figure 8.8):

- The *diencephalon* is a sub-cortical area lying at the base of the forebrain. It includes the dorsomedial nucleus of the

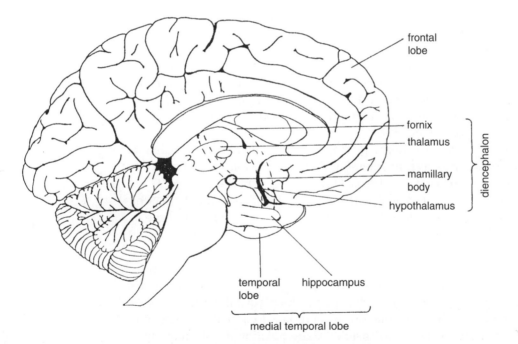

Fig. 8.8 Sagittal section of the brain to show the position of the diencephalon and the medial temporal lobe.

thalamus and the mamillary bodies. This brain area is associated with both anterograde and retrograde amnesia due to decay in storage of memory traces and retrieval problems. Diencephalic amnesia occurs as a result of chronic alcoholism and the associated thiamine deficiency. In Korsakoff's amnesia the frontal lobe is also typically damaged.

- The *medial temporal lobe* and *hippocampus* are associated with severe anterograde loss, characterised by inability to learn and store new material. Temporal lobe amnesia occurs after severe temporal lobe damage due to viral encephalitis and progressive atrophy in Alzheimer's disease. PET scan studies have shown that the hippocampus plays an important role in episodic memory.

Some of the features of temporal lobe amnesia are described in the case study from Wilson & Wearing (1995) given in the section on procedural memory. Further exploration of all memory disorders can be found in Baddeley *et al.* (2002).

Confabulation

Confabulation is the falsification of memory associated with amnesia. It has been called 'honest lying'. *Spontaneous confabulation* is unprovoked and the person may act according to a false memory. There is a failure to suppress currently irrelevant memories which intrude on the present time so that actions or speech are put in the wrong context. For example, an amnesic person, who was a former executive, regularly requested to leave the hospital ward to go to a meeting.

Non-spontaneous confabulations are provoked in answer to a question. Incorrect information, though plausible, is given in the response to questions such as 'Have you seen this before?' or 'How many children do you have?' Both the details and the context of a memory are confused, and the relationship of events in time is disrupted. Confabulation is not a simple loss of memories and it coincides with a loss of insight.

Retrieval in normal memory requires the development of a strategy to activate stored knowledge with particular time and space dimensions, as well as verification of its plausibility and consistency with other information. If there is a loss of these checking procedures there is no insight. Confabulation most frequently occurs in people with frontal lobe lesions. The common features of processing and the anatomical location suggest that confabulation may be a memory impairment with an overlay of dysexecutive syndrome (see Chapter 10).

FUNCTIONAL CONSEQUENCES OF LONG-TERM MEMORY DEFICITS

The inability to recognise objects, faces and landmarks can be the result of long-term memory loss. In daily living, familiar articles in a home setting are the most likely to be recognised. The memory impaired person may place articles in unusual positions in the house, for example a kitchen utensil on a table in the bathroom.

Daily routines are either not activated at the right time or not activated at all. People with severe loss of prospective memory are not able to live independently. Memory for former daily routines and appointments may be intact, except when they involve information or words that are no longer in semantic memory. The timetable for daily or weekly events may not be recalled, for example when to put out the wheelie bin. Parents organising young children need to remember which day a child goes swimming or needs to take dinner money. Personal or family safety may be compromised if the person cannot remember whether the door was locked or the gas was turned off on the cooker. Friends may be upset when social engagements are forgotten.

Memory dysfunction can lead to loss of identity and independence. The phrase 'we are what we remember' expresses clearly the importance of memories of the past to give us a sense of self. People, places and objects, as well as the events we have experienced, are part of autobiographical memory. A vase on a shelf or a postcard in a drawer can vividly retrieve the memory of a holiday in the distant past with all the associated people and events. When this memory has gone, the sense of loss for the family and friends, as well as the person, is great. Social interaction with family and friends is difficult when the person cannot talk about the events they have enjoyed together in the past and this leads to a loss of self-esteem. The identification of a spared work or leisure skill may restore self-esteem and provide motivation for further memory training.

Watching TV, visiting the cinema and reading the newspaper cannot be enjoyed if the storyline cannot be followed. Sport enthusiasts cannot remember what happened in the last game. Spared procedural memory retains the ability to perform sporting activities learnt in the past, although memory aids are needed for the parts of the activity that rely on semantic memory, for example scoring.

Memory loss may have minimum effect on some people who are well supported by family and carers. For others, the loss may have widespread effects on daily living, social interaction, leisure pursuits and employment. After brain damage, some people deny that they have a memory problem because their new environment makes few demands on memory. In degenerative conditions, the deterioration of memory may be gradual and difficult to separate from other cognitive changes.

SUGGESTIONS FOR ASSESSMENT AND INTERVENTION

Assessment

- Read a short sequence of numbers at the rate of one digit per second and ask the person to repeat the numbers back in the same order. Increase the number of digits until an error occurs or a maximum of eight digits is reached. Repeat this task, but asking the person to reverse the numbers.

- Observe the person making a telephone call or discuss an article read in the daily newspaper, for example (if meaningful to the person) ask them to find the football scores and weave this back into the conversation later to see if they can remember their team's result.

- Consider the use of multi-task activities within your assessment. Consider an assessment involving making lunch, with hot drink and sandwiches to be prepared simultaneously.

- Consider the impact of the environment where the assessment is occurring, an unfamiliar kitchen within an occupational therapy department may hinder optimal functional performance.

Assessment resources

Standardised assessment tools also measure different types of memory and these include Doors and People (long-term memory), the RBMT (everyday memory) and the COTNAB.

Intervention

- Using an errorless learning approach will help to prevent new learning of mistakes.
- Use repetition and rehearsal with verbal and/or visual cues to aid performance.

- Introduce compensatory strategies to manage the anxiety and frustration caused by memory difficulties, for example set speed dialling buttons on the telephone, an alarm as a prompt to check a diary.
- If appropriate, consider the provision of education and information to the person and their family to increase knowledge and understanding of memory impairments.
- Establish a diary system as a compensatory technique. The person is prompted to complete it (if able) and family and friends can add information. Use this as a prompt and not a test to help orientation, for example, 'I see from here that your wife visited last night and you went out for a coffee'. Encourage others to do the same.

Sources of evidence

Evans *et al.* (2000) present experiments conducted in nine centres in Europe and one centre in Argentina, comparing errorless learning to trial and error methods for those with memory deficits. The results support the use of errorless learning for tasks which facilitate implicit memory for learned material, for example recalling names. In contrast, the approach was no more beneficial than trial and error when explicit recall of novel tasks was required, for example learning a route. Furthermore, those with more severe memory impairments benefited to a greater extent using errorless learning.

Whilst not specific to memory impairments, Niemeier *et al.* (2005) present preliminary results indicating that people with brain injury may benefit from education and information even in the acute stages of recovery. A neurobehavioural group intervention, First Steps, has been devised which aims to provide basic information for patients, families and care givers about a range of cognitive impairments associated with traumatic brain injury, teach compensatory strategies, empower individuals and provide a ready reference for discharge. The programme utilises a multidisciplinary approach and can be adapted for people with severe cognitive disabilities.

Summary

1. Working memory theory is an account of how verbal and visuo-spatial information from the sensory store is held for a

short time, while some active processing for meaning occurs, before passing on to long-term memory. Verbal (speech based) items are rehearsed in the phonological loop. Attention is allocated between the visual and verbal components by a central executive. Items from visual and verbal sources are integrated by the episodic buffer. Information retrieved from long-term memory is processed in working memory before response in speech or action.

2. Deficits in working memory may affect the understanding of speech and written text. Finding the way in a known route and manipulating money for shopping may also be difficult. Competition for the limited resources in working memory for visual and verbal processing leads to difficulty in dual task performance.

3. The structure of long-term memory can be divided into declarative memory for facts and events that are explicitly retrieved, and procedural memory for learnt motor and verbal skills which are implicit and without conscious access. Prospective memory is a store of plans for future action and behaviour which usually have to be activated without external cues.

4. Processing in long-term memory occurs in three stages. The first stage is registration at the time of learning, which depends on the level of processing, elaboration and context. The second stage is retention over time, which is affected by modification and interference from new memories. The third stage is retrieval, which is achieved with or without awareness and is affected by context and mood.

5. Schema theory describes how stored knowledge relating to one situation (object, person, action or event) may be organised. Schemas develop because of experience and they guide top-down processing of incoming information to meet expectations.

6. The main brain areas involved in memory are the diencephalon, the medial temporal lobes and the frontal lobe. The hippocampus in the temporal lobe plays a pivotal role in the integration of memory systems. Long-term episodic and semantic memory can be selectively impaired, while procedural memory is usually spared. The features of amnesia include inability to learn new material, decay of stored memories and retrieval problems.

7. Long-term memory deficits result in loss of identity and independence. Social interaction with family and friends is

severely affected by the loss of episodic memory. Participation in leisure games depends on memory aids for the semantic aspects such as scoring. Employment prospects are poor when the work involves a significant knowledge base. New learning is difficult and this becomes a hurdle in moving to a different job or home environment where novel ways of doing tasks must be learnt.

9 Purposeful Movement and Apraxia

In all the movements we make, patterns of muscle activity are generated in response to commands from the motor centres in the brain. These motor programmes define the force, direction and timing of the muscle activity. The resulting movements are coordinated by sub-cortical areas of the brain. The performance of effective purposeful movements demands additional processing of knowledge of objects and actions associated with their use. The sequence of actions in goal-oriented movement must be planned and then executed in the correct order to reach that goal. Correct matching between the object and the action must occur at each stage in a sequence of actions. A mismatch between an object and the action related to it is seen in performance errors (see Figure 9.1). Working memory selects the relevant environmental cues, and retrieves stored procedural knowledge from long-term memory. Attention is required for monitoring and modifying the actions in response to changing conditions.

People who show poor task performance may have motor and/or sensory deficits, identified by the assessment of sensation, muscle tone, motor patterns and balance reactions. Others, with minimal motor or sensory loss, have difficulties in the execution of goal-oriented movement, particularly when the task uses more than one object. Errors occur when the conceptual knowledge related to objects cannot be integrated with the movements related to their use, for example drinking from a cup must activate reaching and grasping. When conceptual knowledge is intact, errors can occur in the production of movement, if the person cannot carry out what is intended.

Cognition and task performance

Cognition plays a major role in all meaningful and goal directed activities.

• Sensation and perception

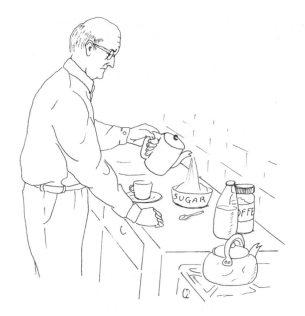

Fig. 9.1 Purposeful movement – performance error.

Visual and auditory information about the position and movement of objects is incorporated into the planning of movement. The manipulation of objects includes tactile feedback about their weight and the strength of grip required. We are aware of a mismatch between planning and perception if we pick up a carton of juice that is nearly empty when expecting it to be full, or walk up an escalator that is not working. Perceptual processing monitors the changing features of the environment during movement and errors are corrected based on the feedback from sensory input. Walking on different surfaces and around obstacles involves tactile input from the soles of the feet. The balance of the body is maintained by the integration of this touch sensation with vision and with proprioceptive information from the muscles and the joints. Visuo-spatial perception allows us to orient the body in the correct position and direction as we move around in space.

- Memory and learning
  Skilled activities and motor routines are developed with practice and stored in procedural memory. When the learned routine for riding a bicycle or driving a car is activated, the sequence of movements is performed automatically. During the progress along a route, declarative knowledge is retrieved

into working memory for the recognition of landmarks recalled from occasions in the past. Remembering to act at some time in the future depends on prospective memory. The action may be triggered by a prompt, for example seeing a post-box when a letter needs to be posted, or we rely on our own strategy for initiating the action.

- High level executive functions
The executive functions enable us to deal with novel situations and challenges. Goals must be formulated and movements planned before initiation. The changing demands during the progress of an activity involve flexible problem solving to reach the goal. Self-awareness and insight play a major role in purposeful activity.

- Emotion
Emotion has an effect on our attention to the task in hand and directly affects the quality of movement. In choosing how to act, incoming sensation and perceptual processing are integrated with our values and our emotional state at the time. Consider the example of a parent or carer walking to meet a child from school. The mother may meet a neighbour who has been ill and wishes to chat. Emotional factors guide the parent's decision whether to stop and talk or to be on time for the child at school. There is evidence that the pre-frontal area assesses the emotional quality of stimuli and influences decision making in movement.

In the OTPF (AOTA, 2002), cognition in task performance is considered as process skills under the following headings:

> *Energy* includes pacing and attention for the planning and progress of a task to completion.
> *Knowledge* recognises the importance of recall of the procedure from memory, together with the selection of the appropriate tools and materials required.
> *Temporal organisation* includes initiation, sequencing and termination of a task.
> *Organising space and objects* requires object recognition and spatial ability to search and navigate within the environment.
> *Adaptation* is an executive function that supports the ability to modify actions in response to changes in the environment.

Programmes for action

In the 1970s, psychologists who were interested in the acquisition of motor skills adopted an information processing approach to normal motor behaviour. The term *motor programme* or *engram*, was introduced to describe a stored action memory for a particular movement. The early description of the motor programme was a set of motor commands that execute movement. The motor programme specified not only which muscles are active but also the direction, force and timing of the muscle activity. One problem with this original definition of a motor programme is that it does not account for the execution of a particular movement by different groups of muscles. For example, you can write your signature using different muscle groups.

Activity

Sign your name on a small piece of paper using the fingers and thumb to move the pencil. Then sign your name on a wall mounted board using the muscles of the shoulder and the elbow. The signature is the same, even though different muscle groups have been used in each case.

The motor programme for a simple ballistic movement is programmed before the start. If you press a computer key or throw a piece of paper into a waste basket, once you have started there is no chance of changing the movement. This is known as open loop movement (see Figure 9.2a). Accuracy can be improved in open loop movement so there must be some option for change in the motor programme before the start of the action.

Most of our actions take longer, and we do make changes during the progress of the movement in response to feedback. In pouring water from a kettle into a cup, the movement is modified as it proceeds in response to the weight of the kettle (proprioceptive feedback), and to the level of the water in the cup (visual feedback). This is known as closed loop movement (see Figure 9.2b).

The original concept of a motor programme was extended into a *schema* which incorporates the perceptual as well as the motor components of movement. Schema theory proposed that knowledge of the component actions in a daily living task is organised into a family of schemas. These are activated in a particular order

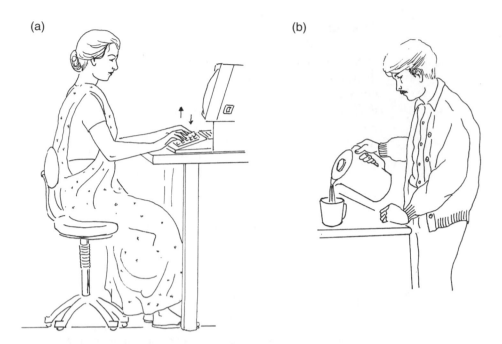

Fig. 9.2 a) Open loop ballistic movements; b) Closed loop movement with feedback.

to reach the goal. The knowledge for a routine activity is organised into a hierarchy of all the action schemas involved. A high level or 'parent' schema defines the goal of the action. Low level or 'child' schemas define the component actions to achieve the goal. A low level schema can be called a sub-schema. Figure 9.3 outlines the organisation of a schema for making a hot drink.

Schema theory suggests that a schema for a specific movement pattern grows with practice in different situations. This supports the value of variable practice in the early stages of learning. A schema for reaching and grasping is strengthened by practice of all the activities that incorporate this movement pattern. Schema theory also supports the principle of normal movement approach, used widely in physical rehabilitation, which incorporates the facilitation of normal movement patterns in all daily living activities.

A high level schema has a set of triggering conditions for activation. When the wrong high level schema is triggered, intention errors are made. We experience this goal switching when we arrive at the supermarket when our intention was to go to the Post Office. During the progress of complex movements, there are transition points from one sub-schema to the next and there is an option of switching to a different one in response to changes in

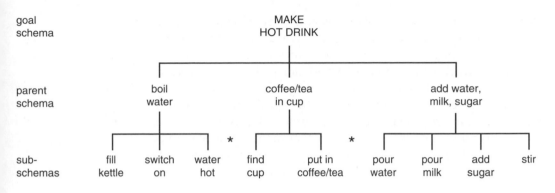

* transition point

Fig. 9.3 Hierarchy of action schemas.

environmental input. Errors occur frequently at transition points from one sub-schema to the next. Boiling the kettle is followed by inserting the tea or coffee into a cup. An omission error at this transition point can lead to pouring water into an empty cup with no tea or coffee. Other errors at this point in a sequence may be repetitions, intrusion of irrelevant actions and actions made in relation to the wrong object.

> **Activity**
>
> Make a list of action errors you make in different situations, for example washing and dressing, meal preparation, leaving the house to go to work, driving, or walking to the shops. Compare your list with others in a group. Are there individual differences? When do action errors occur more frequently?

Similar errors are made by people with cerebral damage, particularly perseveration (repetition of action) at a transition point, when there is inability to move on to the next action sub-schema in the sequence.

Mental practice

Mental imagery can be broadly described as the reproduction of a sensation, object, person or a sequence of events as if it was reality. We can all imagine the details of a scene from a holiday and the events that occurred on that day. We can also use imagery to recall and rehearse a skilled physical activity without doing any movements. Neuropsychologists have debated the relation between perception and imagery and there is some agreement that they share the same processing. The advantage of mental practice is now recognised in sport, music and dance. It is widely believed that the rate of skill acquisition can be significantly improved when added to physical practice, compared with physical practice alone. It is interesting to speculate whether mental practice can be used successfully in rehabilitation. Many people retain the ability to imagine movements mentally in the acute and chronic stage post-stroke.

Bell & Murray (2004) reviewed the studies of the effect of mental practice on improvement of upper limb motor performance after stroke. In most of these studies, subjects engaged in mental prac-tice of upper limb movements presented as a ten-minute audio-tape. Control groups listened to a tape of stroke information or performed physical practice alone. The results showed that the use of mental practice improved the scores on standardised scales for upper limb function although the number of subjects was small and some results were not statistically significant. The authors concluded that mental practice has the potential to widen the scope of intervention and to improve outcomes. However, guide-lines need to be developed on the frequency, length, format and content of this approach.

Models of praxis

Praxis means movement and derives from the Greek for 'doing'. In this instance, it refers to the doing of volitional, goal-directed and purposeful movement. Whilst apraxia is viewed primarily as a cognitive disorder, praxis is a complex interplay between motor, sensory, perceptual and cognitive processes. Our understanding of the production of purposeful movement is enhanced through the exploration of models of praxis. There are two main types of model: neuroanatomical models, seeking to locate the parts of the brain responsible for praxis; and processing models, identifying the levels of processing involved.

Neuroanatomical model

In 1905, Liepmann was the first person to identify a specific motor planning and praxis network within the brain. He first postulated the role of the left hemisphere, especially the left parietal lobe, as dominant for purposeful movement as well as language. The left parietal lobe projects to the left frontal motor areas for movements of the right (dominant) side of the body and via the corpus callosum for the left (non-dominant) side (see Figure 9.4a). The early neuroanatomical model of praxis outlined a system for integration of:

- The left parietal lobe, which stores semantic (conceptual) knowledge of objects and action plans related to their use with
- The motor areas in the frontal lobes, which execute the correct spatial and temporal features of gestures and object-oriented movements

Liepman offered a hierarchical model of the components of the action system (see Figure 9.4b). The specific perceptual processing of sensory information entering the brain accesses the store of action memories related to the concept of movements, called movement formulae. These movement formulae include the motor programme, together with the purpose, plan and sequencing of the action. A movement formula then accesses the innervatory patterns for the muscles which execute the movement. In later

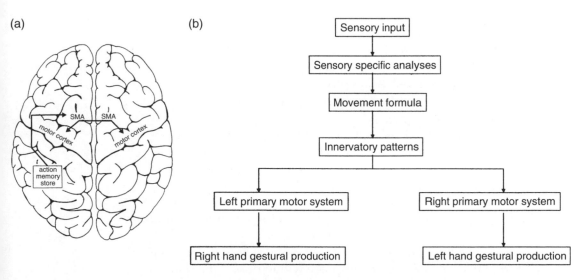

Fig. 9.4 Liepman's models of praxis: a) Anatomical model, SMA – supplementary motor area; b) Hierarchical stages in processing.

accounts by Liepmann, the movement formula was composed of two distinct components: one for action semantics (the idea or concept) and the other for the action plan.

As our understanding has developed, the critique of this model is that it is oversimplified, as there is a need to distinguish between different sensory inputs and also to explain the role of stored motor programmes. Later models of praxis have described parallel processing rather than a hierarchy. Nonetheless, it was Liepmann who first highlighted a movement disorder associated with the use of tools and objects. He also distinguished between the idea and the execution of purposeful movement.

Definition of gestures

Recent studies of praxis in neuropsychology have investigated the production of meaningful gestures. The results of these studies have shown that selective impairment of different types of gestures can occur. There are two main types of gesture production:

1. *Imitation* In this type, the subject copies gestures that are made by the examiner, for example imitation of the movements for combing the hair. The imitation by the subject may be done at the same time, or after an interval of time.
2. *Pantomime* In this case the subject is asked to demonstrate a particular gesture, for example by responding to the command, 'Show me how you would comb your hair'. The command is then followed by the subject performing a mime of the action of hair combing. This type demonstrates the ability of a person to generate a gesture from memory. The term 'pantomime' relates to the original definition of the word as 'a show without words'.

Gestures performed by imitation and by pantomime may or may not involve objects. When an object is held in the hand, the gesture is known as *transitive*, for example if the comb is held in the hand during pantomime, the gesture is transitive. Other gestures do not involve objects and these are known as *intransitive*. Examples are pantomime without the objects, or socio-cultural hand gestures, like a salute or wave goodbye.

Neuro-imaging studies have supported the role of the parietal and frontal lobes in the left hemisphere within praxis, but there is evidence to suggest the involvement of the right hemisphere and also sub-cortical locations. Haaland *et al.* (2000) investigated the neural representations of purposeful movements in people with apraxia and found 8% of their apraxic cohort had right hemisphere strokes. Hanna-Pladdy *et al.* (2001) found that participants with either left or right hemisphere strokes made more errors than a control group when asked to perform gestures, but the two hemispheres showed different types of errors. Only those with left hemisphere strokes showed errors in performing intransitive socio-cultural gestures, like waving goodbye. The same study group demonstrated a role for sub-cortical structures in the brain for the production and execution of tool-based gestures. These studies support the notion that there is a widespread neural praxis network within the brain and the ability to perform meaningful movements is not exclusive to the left parietal lobe.

Processing model

Studies of praxis in cognitive neuropsychology have identified modules of processing in series and in parallel, from auditory (to command) and visual (by imitation) inputs, to output in action. To date there have been few studies of the processing of tactile input from objects. A model of the stages of processing developed by Roy & Square (1994) and outlined in Roy (1996) is shown in Figure 9.5. Three stages of processing are described, but these are not in a hierarchy and stages can be bypassed. The three stages are:

- *Sensory/perceptual system*, which makes a distinction between visual, auditory and object information demonstrated by performance in different types of gesture.
- *Conceptual system* is the semantic system for knowledge of object function and the movements related to their use. The output from the first level accesses this stored knowledge of actions associated with objects and with socio-cultural gestures, for example waving goodbye.
- *Production system* organises and controls response selection and generates the correct innervatory patterns for the movements.

In the model shown in Figure 9.5, 'P' stands for pantomime routes and 'I' for imitation. A person who is able to do imitation is demonstrating that they are still able to process visual/gestural information. Imitation of gestures is divided into concurrent imitation (CI) and delayed imitation (DI), which rely on different memory structures.

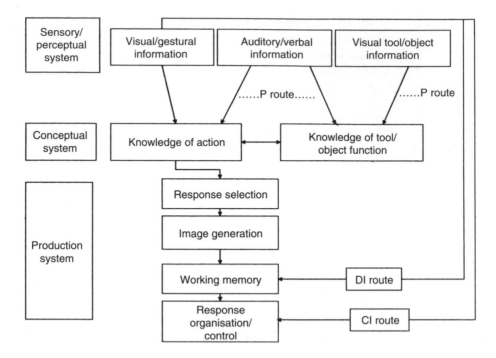

Fig. 9.5   Roy & Square model of praxis based on Roy, Chapter 11 in Elliott & Roy (eds), 1996.

The CI route involves a person performing a task concurrently with the examiner, for example both mime the act of hair combing at the same time. In this case, visual/gestural information accesses directly the response organisation and control stage. This is the only possible route for someone with impaired working memory.

The DI route is used when the person relies on someone else performing the movement, for example an examiner mimes combing the hair and the person copies the gesture later. In using the DI route, the subject needs to store the movements in working memory before imitation on completion of the demonstration. A person who is unable to pantomime a gesture from long-term memory is able to perform delayed imitation of gestures via working memory.

Returning to the model shown in Figure 9.5, the early stages of processing are associated with analysing in parallel: visual/gestural information; auditory input from commands; and visual tool/object input. The next stage involves integration with semantic processing of knowledge of object function and the actions associated with their use. The later stages include response selection and/or image generation, which translate the conceptual knowledge into action. The final stage is the organisation and control of the response, which includes movement sequencing and coordination.

Understanding apraxia

Definitions

The most cited definition of apraxia is from Geschwind (1975), who described the apraxias as disorders of the execution of learned movement in the absence of weakness, incoordination, sensory loss, incomprehension or inattention to commands. However, there are difficulties with this definition as it is based on exclusion criteria and therefore lists disorders that are not found in apraxia.

Apraxia has also been defined as a disorder affecting the ability to pantomime or imitate gestures (Roy & Square, 1994), which helps to qualify the impact of the impairment. Within occupational therapy there is further confusion as the terms dyspraxia and apraxia are often used interchangeably. Ayres (1985) reports that there is a distinction to make between apraxia and dyspraxia, stating that apraxia is a disorder of learned movement and therefore occurs in adults with acquired neurological disorders; the praxis ability was once present and now it is absent (hence the prefix 'a'). This tends to be a disorder affecting the conceptual or production stages of volitional movement as described in the conceptual-production system model previously. In contrast, dyspraxia is a disorder of new learning of motor patterns and sequences, therefore referring to children who have difficulties acquiring praxis skills (hence the prefix 'dys'). Dyspraxia is often viewed as a disorder affecting the sensory stage of volitional movement, hence the development of sensory integration techniques when working with children.

The neuropsychological literature consistently uses the term apraxia when discussing impairment of volitional movement in adults with acquired brain injury and as this is the focus of this book, the term apraxia will be used throughout this chapter. The distinction goes beyond semantics. If a person has previously learned motor patterns and praxis ability, this may be harnessed within their rehabilitation, for example using mental imagery. On the other hand, the focus of intervention for children with developmental difficulties is sensory integration to enhance new learning.

Different types of apraxia

Geschwind (1975) refers to multiple apraxias and there are many types that are debated and defined within the literature, including bucco-facial, constructional, dressing, gait, gaze, limb and speech apraxia. The term apraxia is applied to each of these disorders, many of which are unrelated in their origin. Concha (1987) separates constructional apraxia as a spatial deficit with an added problem of planning and initiating movements. Dressing apraxia has been challenged as a distinct type. In a review of the literature on dressing ability after stroke (Walker & Walker, 2001) it was concluded that the loss of ability to dress may originate in a language deficit, disorders of visual perception and body scheme, or unilateral neglect. The difficulty in dressing is the functional manifestation of the impairment. Both bucco-facial and limb apraxia present as the inability to make meaningful movements of the face or the limbs respectively. Nevertheless, there is reason to separate bucco-facial from limb apraxia on the grounds of the contribution of the limbic system to the innervations of the facial muscles, whose movements are largely associated with the expression of emotion.

Two main types of apraxia, *ideational* and *ideomotor*, will be described.

Ideational apraxia

Ideational apraxia has been described as an 'agnosia of usage', which is a loss of the knowledge of the use of objects. This definition can be mapped onto the Roy & Square processing model of limb apraxia at the level of the conceptual system (see Figure 9.5). Therefore, ideational apraxia is understood as a disorder in the performance of purposeful movement due to a loss of the conceptual (semantic) knowledge of movement related to objects. This loss of action memories associated with object function means that visual and auditory information related to the function of objects cannot access the conceptual system and the pantomime of gestures is impaired. Imitation remains intact as the visual/gestural route can still be utilised (see Figure 9.5).

Errors are made when using objects and tools in routine task performance and on command. People with ideational apraxia may be able to name and describe the function of objects using visual and tactile information, but they cannot integrate this knowledge with the actions related to their use due to the breakdown at the conceptual level of motor performance.

Ideomotor apraxia

Ideomotor apraxia is defined as a disorder in the selection, timing, and spatial organisation of purposeful movement, causing difficulties in making an organised and controlled motor response. This is a disruption to the production system as defined by Roy & Square (see Figure 9.5).

A person with ideomotor apraxia cannot carry out what is intended and has both impaired pantomime and imitation. This differs from ideational apraxia where imitation is intact. Errors are made when the person is asked to perform object-oriented movements both on verbal command (pantomime) and by copying the examiner (imitation). The spatial and temporal features of the movements are most affected.

There is a debate within the literature about whether ideational and ideomotor apraxia are distinct impairments or overlapping disorders that lie on a continuum of severity. The persisting confusion has been related back to the original work by Liepmann (Hanna-Pladdy & Gonzales Rothi, 2001) because he was the first to make a distinction between the idea and the execution. However, using the conceptual-production system model it is evident that apraxia is caused by breakdowns at several different levels, which are part of the same praxis network. Ideational apraxia relates to breakdown at the conceptual level and ideomotor apraxia refers to the production stage.

Case study (Jackson, 1999)

Mrs B, aged 36 years, had a series of infarcts in the right hemisphere and in the right cerebellar region. She had some residual weakness in the left arm, together with other motor output deficits on the right side. She was right hand dominant. Assessment indicated that poor motor output in the right upper limb was not attributable to a motor or sensory deficit. A screening test for apraxia was used.

Mrs B was able to imitate movements carried out by the occupational therapist, but her movements were clumsy and lacked fluidity. She demonstrated planar errors when performing gestures to verbal command. Errors, including perseveration, body part as object and altered proximity, occurred when demonstrating object use. The use of a hammer was performed as rocking backwards and forwards. A hammering movement was used to demonstrate the use of a saw, when the last action had been the use of a hammer. Similar difficulties with the planar orientation of movements occurred in daily living activities, for example writing and putting on her baby's nappy.

Child care was initially simulated using a doll because she had concerns about her handling skills. It was thought more relevant for her to work with her child as soon as possible to create a realistic setting. Facilitation of normal movement patterns was used to elicit the correct movement patterns in all activities.

Error types

Different error types that are observed within function enable occupational therapists to distinguish apraxia related impairments from other motor impairments, for example hemiplegia. The error types that are produced depend on the level where the breakdown in performance occurs. It must be appreciated that the error types that are observed in function tend to be at the conceptual or production stages because they are the tangible aspect of volitional movement.

In a review of studies of apraxia in neuropsychology over nearly a century, Tate & McDonald (1995) concluded that a definitive account of this impairment remains an enigma. There was a lack of consistency in the features of the action errors described by different authors and a wide range in the number of errors suggested as criteria for the diagnosis. These differences can only be resolved by a consensus of opinion on what constitutes an error, based on detailed analysis and recording of error types (York & Cermak, 1995). Research continues to identify different apraxic error types.

Table 9.1 lists the error types that have been identified to date, together with functional examples associated with each.

Figure 9.6 shows the performance errors of:

1. Using body part as object
2. Action in the wrong plane

In occupational therapy, the ability of an individual with a neurological impairment to perform goal-directed movement is assessed within functional activities. When errors occur that cannot be explained by the exclusion factors cited by Geschwind (1975), the term apraxia should be considered. It should be noted that errors may be compounded by other factors, such as the role

Table 9.1 Error types observed during volitional movement.

Error type	Functional example
Omissions	A step within a task is left out, for example does not put paste on the toothbrush
Difficulty terminating movements	Continues to stir the coffee for a prolonged period
Repetitions	Washes the same body part again
Disturbances to order of movements in sequence	Attempts to pour the milk from the bottle without removing the lid
Difficulties coordinating limbs in time and space	May overshoot when reaching for the kettle or have difficulty with tasks that require the use of both arms
Perseveration	Performs the same movement in two consecutive activities, for example stirs the coffee, then stirs the sugar instead of spooning action
Performance in wrong plane	May wave goodbye with a flat hand
Using body part as object	Uses hand to comb hair
Verbalise performance without completing	Able to talk through the steps required but not able to complete the actions
Poor performance to verbal command, for example, 'Show me how you would butter the toast'	Presses the butter into the toast with a knife instead of spreading it
Mismatching object to action	Attempts to comb hair with a tube of sweets

of the environment. Some people can function within their home environment but may make errors when asked to perform the same activities in an unfamiliar one, for example wash and dress by the hospital bed. Moreover, some people are able to use objects and tools, but struggle with socio-cultural gestures such as waving goodbye to a relative.

Goldenberg & Hagmann (1998) developed a functional assessment that can be readily used within clinical practice. The subject is required to perform three activities: spreading margarine, putting on a T-shirt and brushing teeth. Each task is broken down into component parts. The rater is required to make notes at each step of the activity and identify if an error is made in relation to the selection of objects, the movements, or the sequence. The errors are

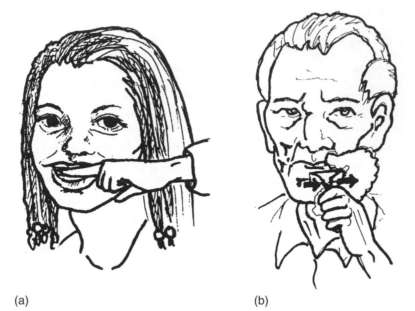

(a)   (b)

Fig. 9.6 Action errors: a) Brushing the teeth, body part as object; b) Shaving, action in the wrong plane.

classed as either reparable or fatal. The therapist only intervenes if a fatal error occurs, that is if the person is unable to carry on with the activity. The authors reported significant inter-rater reliability in assessing for fatal errors. This type of assessment gives information about where the task performance is breaking down and proves to be a useful tool to aid intervention planning. It does not allow for the assessment of apraxia which is not associated with the use of tools and objects.

A different approach to the assessment of apraxia is the analysis of gestures. This can be useful as a screening tool in clinical practice. Zwinkels *et al.* (2004) and Almeida *et al.* (2002) developed assessments using subtests to separate transitive (with tool or object) and intransitive gestures. These tests involved a specific set of activities, for example using a spatula or tweezers, or signalling the 'OK' sign, although the latter is not universal. In transitive gestures, the subject must imitate the use of the object and then demonstrate the actual use. The analysis of the performance of gestures allows us to distinguish different levels of impairment in apraxia. Roy & Square categorised eight major levels with different praxic performance patterns, based on the ability to pantomime and imitate gestures, both concurrent and delayed.

Butler (2002) concluded that tests can identify people as apraxic because they elicit different aspects of the disorder. She argues, however, that it may be more clinically relevant to consider functional and behavioural indices in activities of daily living rather than strive for test scores within the assessment process.

> **Activity**
>
> Mr MFP, aged 72, is a film producer who had an extensive middle cerebral artery infarct. On admission to the rehabilitation unit, he did not have independent sitting balance and he had no functional use of his right arm. He was unable to speak or understand verbal instruction. Standardised tests were inappropriate and observation of function was used. When attempting to eat slices of banana, he would overshoot when reaching for them. He occasionally took his hand to his mouth without a piece of banana present, or when present he would bring the food to his mouth with his wrist in flexion and hand in pronation.
>
> Using the information from this case study, discuss how you might identify the level(s) where the breakdown in performance occurs for Mr MFP, using the conceptual-production model of Roy & Square.

FUNCTIONAL CONSEQUENCES

People with apraxia make errors when performing activities using objects and tools. Errors are reduced in a familiar environment, for example brushing the teeth in the bathroom at home. Single actions, such as putting a plug into a socket or turning on the tap, may be done fluently, but the situation changes when an activity involves sequencing and the use of more than one object (see Figure 9.7). The component actions in a sequence may be in the wrong order, or a stage may be omitted, for example stirring a coffee mug with no water in it, or two parts of the sequence may be blended together. Miller (1986) described the omission of a crucial step and mismatch of object and action in a man with apraxia. He attempted to pour himself a drink of orange squash by first pouring without unscrewing the top of the bottle, then continuing to pour with the cap removed, and finally emptying it into the water jug instead of the glass.

Sequencing in dressing is usually unique to the individual. Some people dress the lower body before the upper body and vice versa. In apraxia, sequencing errors may lead to underclothes being put on top of outer clothing. Playing a musical instrument requires

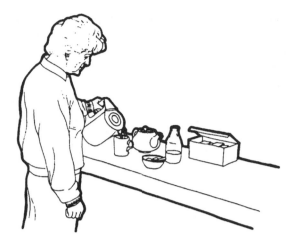

Fig. 9.7 Task using multiple objects.

sequencing of the notes and using a computer demands a serial order of pressing the function keys.

Perseveration of an action may occur, particularly at transition points from one action to another in a sequence. A teacup may be placed on a saucer, and then the action is repeated with the teapot on a saucer. In eating, overshooting may occur in reaching to pick up pieces of food on a plate and the spoon may be held upside down when eating from a bowl.

Some apraxic people can perform object based activities but they struggle with socio-cultural gestures. A hand offered in greeting may not result in the person grasping and shaking it. This may be due to the inability to recognise the gesture (conceptual error) or the person being unable to produce the movement in response (production error).

Some people with apraxia are unaware of the errors they are making and are in danger of causing accidents, such as leaving the gas unlit on the cooker. In other cases, the person is aware of the errors being made but can do nothing to correct them. They may be wrongly labelled as confused.

In the familiar home environment, there may be no problems with routine tasks that can be completed automatically. When the attention demands increase, the movements lack fluency and look clumsy. This can be a source of irritation to the individual and the family. In the absence of other problems, the person with apraxia can function reasonably well at home, but safety is at risk.

SUGGESTIONS FOR ASSESSMENT AND INTERVENTION

Assessment

- Use activities that require transitive (tool-based) and intransitive (socio-cultural) gestures.
- Ascertain if a person is able to pantomime and imitate (both concurrent and delayed). Ask them to perform an activity to verbal command with and without the object present, and then use a photograph as a cue (also helpful if communication skills are impaired). Relate this information to the conceptual-production model of praxis to determine the level(s) of breakdown in performance.
- Observe function within a naturalistic environment whenever possible.
- Document the types of errors observed and note if the person is able to overcome them (reparable) or if the errors are fatal (that is the therapist needs to intervene to aid continuation of the task).
- Consider the different stages of goal-directed movement and observe at which stage the breakdown may be occurring, for example sensory/perceptual, conceptual or production stages.

Assessment resources

Goldenberg & Hagmann (1998) report on an assessment using daily living tasks to test for error types. Zwinkels *et al.* (2004) and Almeida *et al.* (2002) utilised subtests to separate transitive and intransitive gestures, which are useful as screening tools in clinical practice. Standardised assessment tools also measure apraxia within the component sections and these include the LOTCA and the AMPS. Details of the AMPS can be found in AMPS Traning Manual, Wiltshire, UK.

Intervention

- Carry out intervention sessions within the naturalistic environment wherever possible and use items within the environment for non-verbal cues.
- Intervention must be task specific and the activity must be a real priority for the client.
- Consider using hand-over-hand guidance or normal movement techniques if the breakdown of performance is at the sensory or conceptual level.

- Consider if delayed imitation or concurrent imitation is appropriate for the individual person.
- Use an errorless learning approach and repetition, intervening before errors occur to facilitate learning and to improve function.
- Teach a person and their family the concept of activity analysis and chaining; they may wish to transfer this technique to other priority activities and take control of their own rehabilitation.
- Minimise the amount of verbal cues – there is a high association with apraxia and communication difficulties.

Sources of evidence

Edmans *et al.* (2001) and Jackson (1999) provide guidelines devised from clinical experience and the evidence within the literature. They suggest using chaining, activities in context, error recognition and normal movement within intervention, but the choice of strategy must be guided by clinical reasoning, which includes knowledge of the impairment. Donkervoort *et al.* (2001) conducted a single-blind randomised control trial investigating the efficacy of strategy training, that is teaching compensatory strategies, with a control group receiving usual occupational therapy. They concluded that participants in the strategy training group improved more in observed performance of ADL than patients in the control group, after the eight-week treatment, but with only a small to medium effect and no significant differences at the five-month follow-up review.

Goldenberg *et al.* (2001) looked at the longer-term effectiveness of direct training methods, including verbal and physical prompts at critical stages of an activity, and concluded that direct training induced a significant reduction in the number of errors and assistance required. Furthermore, the training effects were largely preserved at the three-month follow-up review, although the therapeutic gains were restricted to the specific activity restored and did not extrapolate to other activities.

Summary

1. Single actions involve the activation of stored motor programmes which specify the direction, force and timing of muscle activity. In goal-oriented movement, action memories are organised into a hierarchy of schemas which are activated

in serial order to reach the goal. Action errors frequently occur at transition points from one sub-schema to the next.

2. Mental imagery can be used to recall and rehearse learned skilled movement. This process of mental practice has been shown to facilitate performance in sports activities and has the potential to improve outcomes in rehabilitation.

3. Liepman's neuroanatomical model of praxis linked the performance of skilled purposeful movements to the left hemisphere. Action memories stored in the left parietal lobe project to the frontal motor areas for the execution of movements. Recent research has demonstrated that praxis is not exclusive to the left parietal lobe and involves a complex network in many different parts of the brain, including sub-cortical areas.

4. The conceptual-production system model of limb praxis developed by Roy & Square identifies three stages to produce purposeful movement: sensory/perceptual, conceptual (semantic) and production systems. Apraxia is a cognitive disorder that affects the ability to generate the idea of a movement and/or execute a purposeful movement. Ideational and ideomotor apraxias are different but interrelated types of apraxia caused by breakdown at different levels within the praxis network.

5. The exploration of the performance of gestures can be used to assess the level of impairment in apraxia. Some apraxic individuals can imitate gestures but cannot pantomime their actions from memory. Others can perform transitive gestures when an object is present but not intransitive gestures. The error types observed within function enable occupational therapists to distinguish apraxia from motor impairments such as hemiplegia.

10 Executive Functions

For a large part of the day we function on 'autopilot'. Well-established routines, such as making a cup of coffee and driving the car are triggered by the environmental cues and require little of our attention. Your habitual routine for leaving home to go to college or to work probably involves closing the door, checking you have the door key and your bag, and walking a particular route to the station. On Saturday, you may find yourself going through the same routine when you intended to go by bus to the supermarket. In non-routine behaviour, procedures which are not relevant must be inhibited and attention must now be sustained until we achieve the new goal. Novel situations require choices and decisions about what to do and how to do it (see Figure 10.1).

The term *executive function* refers to a range of high level cognitive processes which combine to set goals and to make choices in novel situations. These processes all act to verify whether an activity is appropriate for the current situation. Executive processes regulate action and behaviour by allocating cognitive resources to searching, matching, deciding, monitoring and evaluating.

The pre-frontal cortex has been implicated in the operation of the executive functions, based on evidence from the clinical features of people with frontal lobe lesions and neuro-imaging studies of both normal subjects and patients. Luria (1966) first introduced the term 'frontal lobe syndrome' for the characteristic changes in behaviour resulting from frontal lobe damage. The early clinical accounts described wide-ranging changes in personality. Later clinical studies emphasised the effect on decision making as well as personality. Frontal lobe damage can lead to problems in carrying out tasks that require initiation, planning and organising, or may even result in the complete avoidance of any non-routine activity. Duncan (1986) noted that a common theme in frontal lobe lesion is the disorganisation of activity, which may be expressed across memory, language, movement or problem solving, with failure to achieve known goals. The cluster of symptoms observed in patients with damage to the frontal lobe is now known as *dysexecutive syndrome*.

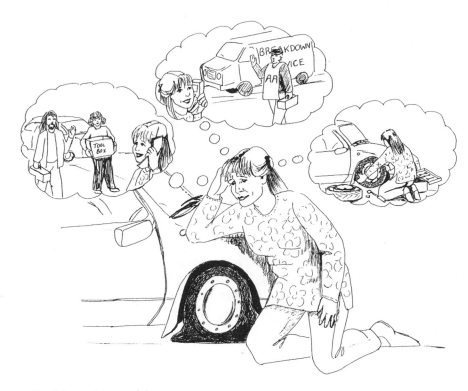

Fig. 10.1 Flexible problem solving.

What are the executive functions?

Executive functions are the higher order cognitive skills for performance of novel goal-directed actions and behaviour. They are coordinated by the frontal lobe, which sends out and receives information from most cortical and some sub-cortical areas. A major role of executive processes is to coordinate and monitor the cognitive system as a whole and to allocate cognitive resources appropriately. Neuropsychologists have attempted to partition the executive system into independent components and have investigated dissociations between them, but so far no definitive list has been developed. The separate executive functions will be described under headings which relate to the component skills defined in occupational therapy:

- Initiation and termination
- Goal setting

- Planning and organising
- Adaptation and flexibility

Initiation and termination

Activity is either initiated by environmental cues or it is internally generated by decision making. Goal-directed activity, which is focused towards the initiation and termination of a specific task, involves the avoidance of behaviour that is cued by the environment. The inability to suppress this activity is seen in laboratory tests when a person with a frontal lobe lesion is asked to copy shapes. The results are incomplete and repetition of the same shape occurs even when the stimulus shape has changed.

In non-routine activity, the suppression of environmentally cued action depends on the inhibition of automatic processing and the maintenance of sustained attention (see Chapter 7). Automatic processes are fast and they are difficult to modify. Controlled processes are relatively slow and capacity limited, but they are flexible when circumstances change.

The Stroop effect is a classic demonstration of interference between automatic and controlled processing. In this test, the stimuli are the names of colour words (red, blue, green, etc.) printed in different colours on individual cards. For example, the word 'red' is presented in red, blue or green colour on separate cards. When each card is presented, subjects are instructed to name the ink colours as rapidly as possible and they are not required to read the word. The results show that subjects name the ink colour much faster if it matches the word itself (the word 'red' written in red colour) than if it does not match (the word 'red' written in blue colour). The presence of the words interferes in the colour naming task. The subjects read the words automatically even though they are not required to do so. The interference leads to a delay in naming the colour. Reading the word is automatic, while identifying the colour is attention dependent.

Interference occurs if we buy a new mobile phone or CD player with function keys in different positions from our previous model. We find ourselves pressing keys in positions corresponding to the well learnt routine of the earlier model. After practice, a new routine is established and this becomes automatic.

A study of initiation and response inhibition was made by Burgess & Shallice (1996). The subjects were in two groups: one group with frontal lobe lesions and the other with posterior lesions. The subjects were presented with a sentence with the last word missing. An example is, 'He mailed a letter without a . . . .' This sentence offers a strong cue for the word 'stamp'. Two conditions were investigated:

1. *Response initiation* – when the subjects were asked to produce a word that completed the sentence.
2. *Response inhibition* – when the subjects were asked to produce a word which made no sense at all in the context of the sentence.

Those with frontal lobe lesions showed a delay in initiating the response in the first condition, taking longer to complete the sentence compared to those with posterior lesions. In the response inhibition, condition the people with frontal lesions again took longer and frequently gave words that made sense when they were asked for nonsense. They were unable to inhibit the automatic response. The results showed no relationship between the measures of initiation and inhibition, which suggests that they are separate components of executive processing. This study has been developed into the Hayling Sentence Completion Test for executive functions.

The lack of response inhibition is often seen during the assessment of persons with frontal lobe damage. Objects placed near to them are grasped and used even when they are told not to do so. This is known as *utilisation behaviour*. In one recorded situation, the subject picked up a pack of cards present on the table and dealt them out correctly for the number of people in the room when he had been asked to do something else. Inability to inhibit automatic processes is also seen as distractibility after frontal lobe damage.

Goal setting

Realistic goal setting depends on the awareness of our own strengths and weaknesses and an estimation of task difficulty. Also, formulating a goal involves thought functions, for example reasoning, which goes beyond the concrete information in the environment and engages in abstract thinking. Abstraction can be assessed using sorting tasks. When people with frontal lesions are asked to sort cards or items that are similar into separate groups, they are unable to abstract a concept or rule for the task. The result is they do not include all the items in the chosen groups and the groupings they choose are not meaningful.

Complex tasks require the setting of sub-goals related to specific steps which must be activated in the correct sequence. An example of this is the overall goal of making a cup of coffee, which has the sub-goals: boil water in a kettle; put coffee in a cup; add milk and sugar. Shallice & Burgess (1991) investigated goal setting in people with frontal lobe damage. Three subjects with head injury were asked to complete three different tasks, each with two components, within the specified time of 15 minutes. The tasks were to dictate a route into an audio recorder, work out simple arithmetic and write down the names of around a hundred pictures of objects. The instructions stated that all tasks should be completed, or a little of each component of each of the tasks. The three subjects with frontal head injury tackled from two to five tasks compared with normal controls who completed nearly all the tasks. One subject made notes for four minutes on the dictation task but never dictated any of it. Another subject looked at the stopwatch seven times but did not switch tasks. Shallice & Burgess claim that the detail of the results cannot be explained on the grounds of retrospective memory impairment and/or lack of motivation. The brain-damaged subjects were unable to develop strategies to achieve sub-goals for the component parts of the task. This test has been developed into the Six Elements Test.

Planning and organising

Effective planning and organising involves the formation of strategies to achieve the desired goal. During the progress of a task, conditions may change and new strategies need to be activated until the goal is reached. Returning to the example of a flat tyre on a car (see Figure 10.1) the goal is to acquire a functional wheel and tyre. This will involve several stages:

- Identify the problem and the solution.
- Formulate a plan and activate strategies to achieve the goal. The plan may be to change the tyre yourself, to call for help from a friend or from a breakdown service.
- Modify the plan if no help is available.

The choice of strategies requires the ability to estimate both task difficulty and the time needed to complete the task. In this example, there are the sub-goals of making phone calls and moving the car to a safe part of the road. The most effective strategy may be to leave the car and go home by bus.

The ability to develop higher order planning to achieve a goal was explored in the Multiple Errands Task devised by Shallice &

Burgess (1991). In this test, three people with frontal lobe lesions and nine control subjects were given instructions to complete eight tasks in a shopping precinct, an environment where unpredictable events can occur. Six of the tasks were related to shopping (for example buy a brown loaf). The seventh task required the person to be in a specific place 15 minutes after starting. For the eighth task, four pieces of information (for example the price of a pound of tomatoes), two of them unrelated to shopping, had to be written on a postcard during the errands. The observers noted qualitatively different performance of the tasks by the three subjects with frontal lobe damage, which reflected poor planning and organisation. Although one of the subjects completed all the tasks satisfactorily, errors in the execution by all three of them were related to both the inability to follow the instructions exactly as given and to devise an effective strategy. The observations of the behaviour of subjects doing the Multiple Errands Test clearly demonstrated the effects of executive deficits on the behaviour of people with frontal lobe damage in real life situations.

A major part of planning is the ability to formulate intentions. Furthermore, the intention needs to be activated at a later date when there is no cue or prompt for the intended action. Shallice & Burgess (1991) suggested that *intention markers* are temporarily created in memory and they are triggered when the relevant situation occurs. They explain the marker as a message that future behaviour is not routine and requires specific action. In this way, executive processes facilitate the realisation of goals and intentions. An example is the forward planning we may do before we leave home in the morning. If we get a phone call from a friend asking us to meet in the evening, the plan for the end of the day now includes taking a train to a different destination after work. The intention marker relates to a particular time in the day and must be activated when we leave work. If the situation changes, for example there is a train drivers' strike, the intention marker must be cancelled and a new response must be formulated.

Adaptation and flexibility

Adaptation has been defined as a change a person makes in his or her response approach when that person encounters an occupational challenge (Christianson & Baum, 1997). If the challenge is a routine task, cues in the environment will trigger a new schema for the change to a different routine. For example, the telephone ringing while you are cooking supper cues the response to go to the phone. Adapting to the new challenge demands termination of cooking in a way that is safe and does not result in burnt food. Furthermore, when the phone call is over, cooking must be initiated at the correct step. This simple example illustrates the role of adaptation in daily activities.

The ability to monitor what is going on in the environment is an important component of flexibility. Self-monitoring requires self-enquiry about how the task is progressing and keeping track of the steps in a sequence. A person with frontal lobe damage is easily distracted and finds it difficult to get back on track, particularly in prolonged tasks with multiple steps.

An early test of flexibility was designed to measure the ability to formulate concepts and to switch from one concept to another. In the Wisconsin Card Sorting Test (Milner, 1963), the subject is asked to sort cards into four piles so that each matches one of four stimulus cards which vary by number, shape and colour (see Figure 10.2). The number of items on the card ranges from one to four; the shape of items is either a triangle, star, cross or circle; and the colour is either red, green, yellow or blue. At first, the cards are sorted by one particular rule, for example red crosses. As each card is placed, the subject is told whether or not the card matches the experimenter's rule. After six successful applications, the experimenter changes the rule either with or without warning to a different stimulus, for example green stars. The subjects with frontal lobe damage find that rule shifting is difficult when the category changes. They show perseveration and continue to sort by the previous rule when it is no longer required and carry on even when told it is wrong.

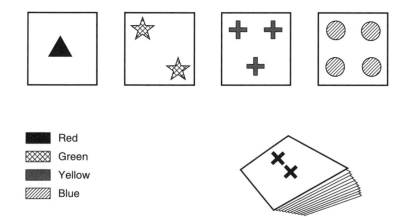

Red
Green
Yellow
Blue

Fig. 10.2 Wisconsin Card Sorting Test, cards presented to the subject. Reproduced with permission from Milner (1963) *Archives of Neurology* 9, 90–100. Copyright 1963, American Medical Association.

More recently, flexibility has been assessed in tests of mental fluency. One of these is the Alternative Uses Test, which asks the subject to think of unusual uses for an everyday object. For example, a newspaper can be read but can also be used to swat flies. People with frontal lobe damage are unable to switch away from the typical use.

Some individuals with frontal lobe damage perform well in desktop tests when only one task is performed in the presence of verbal or visual prompts. The situation changes in daily living when there are no explicit prompts and concurrent tasks must be performed. The person who cannot adapt will meet an occupational challenge with the continuation of rigid behaviour and perseveration of action.

Activity

Discuss the following scenario.

You arrive at the station to catch the train to college or work and find that all the trains have been cancelled due to signal failure. You have a mobile phone and your purse contains two pounds of cash but you left your credit card at home.

List the executive functions that are involved in your subsequent action and behaviour.

Memory and emotion

Many individuals with frontal lobe damage show emotional changes which result in severely disrupted social behaviour. A possible cause may be an inability to integrate knowledge of appropriate behaviour with the consequences of a particular action.

Case study (Eslinger & Damasio, 1985; Saver & Damasio, 1991)

EVR, aged 35 years, was a successful accountant who had bilateral surgical removal of a tumour on the medial frontal lobes. After surgery, he performed normally on IQ tests, the Wisconsin Card Sort test and he was above average on tests of working memory. In the presence of intact cognitive skills, his social conduct was profoundly changed. He behaved without consideration of the consequences of his actions either to himself or to others. He was described as immersed in trivial matters at the expense of more important ones, so that he was unable to make decisions about, for example, what clothes to wear. He was unable to find employment after a series of attempts and was divorced twice. The changes in behaviour may be explained by a disconnection between the knowledge of required behaviour processed in the medial frontal lobes and the actual behaviour activated by the limbic system. This disruption led to responses that had no consideration of the social consequences.

Working memory plays an important role in the evaluation of response options by the manipulation of information retrieved from long-term memory of the same situation in the past. The recall of items from long-term memory also incorporates the knowledge of the positive and negative consequences. This is the basis of adaptation, a performance skill which evaluates alternative behaviours before the execution of a response.

Damasio (1994) formed the hypothesis that the evaluation is guided by a context-linked type of episodic memory with emotional associations, known as *source memory*. Damasio measured the physiological responses that occurred when subjects viewed images with emotional features. A group of subjects with brain damage and normal controls were shown three different types of stimuli: abstract images, countryside scenes and disturbing images. The galvanic skin responses of the control group of subjects showed a marked increase when viewing the disturbing images, but the group who were brain damaged showed a consistent skin response to the three different types of images presented. They could verbally describe the detail in the disturbing pictures but they showed no affective response.

Damasio proposed that somatic markers ('soma' means body) are generated in memory. These markers are brought into working memory when the same situation arises at a later time. The emotional memories then guide the decision about the response to that situation. When there is damage to the pre-frontal cortex, the memories are recalled without the affective content and decisions are then made purely on rational grounds. This is known as the Somatic Marker Hypothesis.

Routine and non-routine behaviour

In daily living, habitual routines that are well established in memory, for example making a cup of coffee, cleaning our teeth, or using a mobile phone, are triggered by the environment and proceed to termination, requiring little of our attention. Non-routine activities require novel patterns of behaviour to be implemented and established skills have to be adapted and organised. Examples of these could include making the coffee in a different coffee maker, or using a new mobile phone with unfamiliar functions. The range of abilities which combine to organise and regulate non-routine activities were described in the first section of this chapter. We will now consider the operation of the executive functions as described in an information processing model (Shallice, 1982). The main feature of the model is the distinction between habitual and novel action routines.

Supervisory attention system

Habitual routines are controlled by organised schemas which are activated in a particular order to reach the goal (see Chapter 9). In the Shallice model, environmental cues trigger a database, which in turn accesses a hierarchy of stored memory representations (known as schemas) for routine activities (see Figure 10.3). Once a schema is activated, it competes with other schemas for dominance in the control of action. If conflict occurs in schema selection then an operation called *contention scheduling* prevents the selection of more than one schema by inhibiting all others. In this way, contention scheduling determines the priority of one set of actions over others.

We will take an example of making a sandwich. The environmental stimulus for this action may be the feeling of hunger or the time on the clock. This triggers a high level schema for making a sandwich.

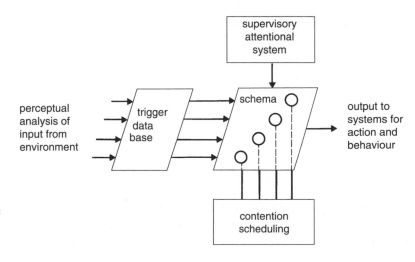

Fig. 10.3 Shallice model, the selection of action schemas (based on Shallice, 1982).

In order to achieve the goal, the task is broken down into a series of smaller sub-routines in a particular order. The first sub-routine is the selection of the bread, butter and a knife, followed by the second sub-routine of spreading the butter on the bread. Preparation of the filling is followed by placing it in the correct position between the two pieces of bread. The final sub-routine is putting the sandwich on a plate and cutting it in half. These sub-routines must be executed in the correct order, for example the filling must not be inserted before the bread is buttered. Shallice proposed that once a high level schema stored in memory is activated, other competing schemas, for example preparing beans on toast, are inhibited. This operation which prevents two activated schemas from being selected was called *contention scheduling*.

Situations do arise when the selection of action by contention scheduling may be inappropriate, and schemas for novel or non-routine behaviour are involved. Then the activation of schemas occurs by the operation of a *supervisory activation system*, SAS, also known as a supervisory attentional system. This system overrides contention scheduling and heightens a schema's level of activation to achieve a novel goal.

The Shallice model identifies three different levels of executive functioning. First, schema selection for habitual action and thought; second, contention scheduling to resolve conflict in schema selection; and third, controlled processing by the SAS. Activation of the Supervisory Attention System is required for the following situations:

- Planning or decision making
- Novel or flexible response
- Error detection and troubleshooting
- Less well learned response
- Potential danger or risk

Pre-frontal cortex

There is evidence that the SAS is located in the most anterior region of the frontal lobe, known as the pre-frontal cortex (PFC). This area regulates non-routine action and behaviour and suppresses strong habitual responses. Functional neuro-imaging studies suggest that the PFC can be divided into the areas described below:

- The lateral pre-frontal cortex is on the lateral surface of the frontal lobe and anterior to the pre-motor area. The lateral pre-frontal cortex selects task relevant information from stored memories in other brain areas, and retains it in working memory for the planning of appropriate action in relation to goals.

- The medial pre-frontal cortex is on the inner aspect of each frontal lobe. The medial frontal cortex is associated with the limbic system, which guides the emotional evaluation of behaviour.
- The anterior cingulate cortex (ACC) is on the medial aspect of the frontal lobe above the corpus callosum. The ACC activates the supervisory attention system when the task requirements differ from the operation of schema by contention scheduling. This serves as a monitoring system and resolves conflict in task requirements.

Return to Chapter 4, Figures 4.8a and b.

Metacognition

Metacognition is our knowledge and beliefs about our own cognitive processes and capacities. It has been called 'knowing what you know'. This knowledge allows us to monitor our own thoughts, speech and actions. Without metacognition we are unable to monitor our changing behaviour or to evaluate strategies for change. The executive functions are inextricably linked with awareness in metacognition, with awareness as the more static component. Loss of awareness leads to inability to detect errors in performance or to anticipate problems and plan strategies. The executive functions are dynamic and operate as a control system for self-monitoring and self-guidance.

Conceptual frameworks for metacognition, based on a hierarchy, have been developed (Sohlberg et al., 1993; Katz & Hartman-Maeir, 1997). Three levels are defined in the hierarchy:

- The lowest level is the cognitive skill for the acquisition and use of information from the environment in order for adaptation to environmental demands. This level involves attention, perception and memory.
- The second level is the executive function for the formulation of realistic goals based on stored plans and routines, and for the development of strategies in flexible problem solving.
- The highest level is metacognitive skill for self-monitoring and self-correcting in the regulation of our actions and behaviour.

At each level, there is feedback down to the lower level (see Figure 10.4, based on Sohlberg et al., 1993).

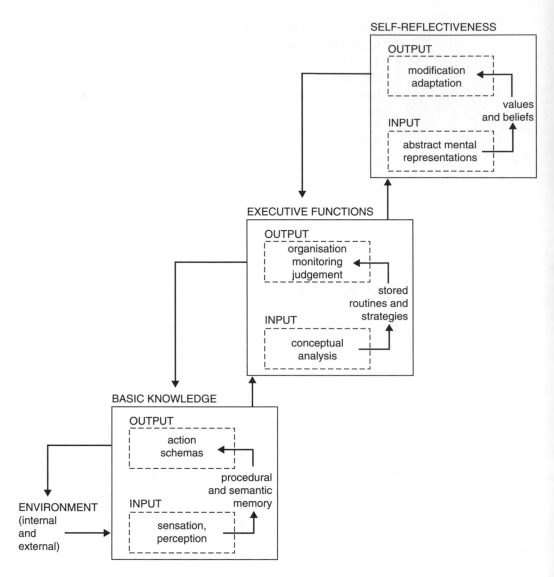

Fig. 10.4 A conceptual framework of the interaction of basic knowledge, executive functions and self-reflectiveness (based on Sohlberg *et al.* 1993).

Dysexecutive syndrome

Dysexecutive syndrome was formerly known as frontal lobe syndrome when Luria (1966) described the frontal lobes as responsible for programming and regulating behaviour. Later accounts described the function of the frontal lobe as the direction and regulation of all the other cognitive systems. Dysexecutive syndrome is now identified by a cluster of symptoms rather than a clearly defined syndrome. Dysexecutive syndrome is commonly seen after traumatic brain injury. People with DES have difficulty in grasping the whole of a complicated state of affairs. He/she may be able to work along routine lines, but cannot master new situations. In task performance, some of the features of DES are similar to apraxia. However, while the ideomotor apraxic person can usually function automatically in a familiar environment, an individual with DES may not be able to organise him/herself to start any activity. Many persons with DES also have memory and attention problems. Pure amnesiacs without DES can still organise themselves by using memory aids; those with DES cannot.

The person with DES may present as apathetic, inflexible and unable to initiate any activity without instructions. On the other hand, he/she may show impulsivity, distractibility and loss of control of ongoing behaviour. Individuals present with a variety of behavioural changes. Loss of affect, lack of motivation, inappropriate social behaviour and lack of insight are all factors which may compound the overall disorganisation of action and behaviour.

Effective planning includes the formulation of a strategy that can be activated at a future time. The estimation of task difficulty and the knowledge of time to complete the task is part of planning. Once activity is initiated, perseveration may occur when contention scheduling is strongly triggered by the environment and the response persists in the absence of control by the executive system. The person may be 'stimulus bound' and unable to change to a different response if the conditions alter.

FUNCTIONAL CONSEQUENCES OF DYSEXECUTIVE SYNDROME

The person with DES may ultimately be unable to organise their own life. Underlying attention deficits lead to loss of orientation to time of day, seasons and situations. When attention is captured, the person with DES may not be able to direct his/her gaze to more than one thing at a time. Verbal instructions are not understood, especially when the response is more than one action. Requests for action need to be given one at a time and with few words. Distractibility interrupts task performance and responses are made to irrelevant stimuli.

Functional problems are compounded when the person returns to the home environment where there is less structure of time and day. The loss of planning ability and self-initiation means that food is not prepared when the person is hungry. This is different from loss of motor initiation when food on a plate is not eaten. Poor initiation may extend to neglect of self-care and failure to communicate with other people. Poor termination means that taps are left running, lights are left on and the door of the refrigerator or freezer is not closed. In task performance there may be repetition of the steps in a sequence, or premature cessation.

In social situations, speech may be verbose, with decreased turn taking and poor topic maintenance. Cooperation with a speech and language therapist is important. Relationships with family and carers may be poor when there is difficulty in regulating social behaviour. Support from the community occupational therapist then becomes essential. The prospects for employment are poor except for occupations based on established routines and sequences.

SUGGESTIONS FOR ASSESSMENT AND INTERVENTION

Assessment

To assess where breakdown in action and behaviour occurs, functional assessments need to be created for the individual. Choose a multi-step task which is non-routine and relevant to the person's current lifestyle. Information from family and friends is useful. The choice of task must also be at the appropriate level of difficulty and one that he or she is likely to complete. At a severe level of impairment, the task may be washing, dressing or organising breakfast. At an intermediate level, the task may be to make a two-course meal, including shopping and budgeting. At a high level of difficulty, the person may plan an outing for a group, or plan to give a presentation on a familiar topic.

A checklist approach, which records performance on each of the individual components of the executive system can be used, such as that constructed by Ylvisacker & Szekeres (1989):

- Realistic goal setting depends on the awareness of the client's own strengths and weaknesses and the estimation of task difficulty. This may be done by asking the client to rate how well he/she thinks the task will be done on a scale of 1 to 10.
  What do you intend to do? Do you think you can do it now? How long will it take?

- Planning is the ability to plan the steps involved to reach the goal. The steps must be executed in the correct sequence to reach the goal. Planning problems lead to impulsive, rigid behaviour with poor time sense.
  Take me through all the steps in doing the activity. Are there any alternative steps?

- Organising is related to carrying out the plan. Part of organising is knowledge of the strategies that may be needed if conditions change. Part of planning may be the appreciation of the situations when assistance is required.
  Do you have the equipment you need? Do you need help from another person?

- Self-initiating is the ability to spontaneously start the task. The level achieved depends on the amount of structure and cueing required for initiation by the client.
  When will you begin the task? Shall I tell you when to start?

- Self-directing is needed to continue with the task once it has been initiated, without seeking reassurance or direction from other people. Self-directing continues until termination at the correct stage in the task.
  Shall I give you prompts during the task? Shall I tell you when the task is going well?

- Self-correcting/self-monitoring. Self-correction is the ability to put something right that has gone wrong. The anticipation of errors requires self-monitoring, so that the course of action is altered to avoid something going wrong. The DES patient may have difficulty in learning from mistakes.
  What problem might you encounter? How would you overcome it?

- Flexible problem solving involves the processing of all the relevant information, and decision making about the most effective solution. Problem solving includes the ability to think of more than one solution to a problem. The DES patient who has learnt new skills cannot transfer them to new situations.
  Can this activity be done in more than one way?

- Self-inhibiting is the basis of turn taking in social interaction. Verbal and non-verbal communication requires self-inhibition for listening and for responding at the appropriate time and place. This component of social skills can be assessed when a client is in a group situation.
  At the end: *Have you achieved your goal for the activity?*

Assessment resources

Standardised assessment tools also measure executive functions, including the BADS and COTNAB. The COTNAB assesses the ability to follow written and verbal instructions. Also, the Cognitive Assessment of Minnesota (CAM) is designed for cognitive screening but may not be readily available in the UK.

Intervention

- Use a collaborative goal-setting approach, encouraging the person to monitor their own progress and work towards setting their own goals if possible. Keep goals relevant and meaningful to the individual.

- Facilitate discussion on error recognition and review performance before, during and after undertaking an activity. For example, how do you think that went? What would you do differently next time? You could use the questions above and note improvements during intervention, for example the number of correct steps identified within the planning phase.

- Work together to establish a daily routine with structure.

Sources of evidence

Norris & Tate (2000) studied the validity of the Behavioural Assessment of Dysexecutive Syndrome (BADS) and expanded upon work from other research groups. They concluded that BADS has greater ecological validity than six other tests of executive function. Cicerone *et al.* (2006) provide a comprehensive analysis of the current evidence for assessment and intervention strategies used with people who have impaired executive functions. Recommendations for future research include exploring the effectiveness of impairment based rehabilitation versus a combined approach for improving activities and participation.

Summary

1. The executive functions initiate and organise actions and behaviour when we are confronted by new situations. The component parts of the executive system have been considered as initiation and termination, goal setting, planning and organising, adaptation and flexibility.

2. Habitual behaviour is activated by environmental triggers which select appropriate stored schemas and inhibit all other conflicting schemas. This is known as contention scheduling. Shallice proposed a supervisory attention system (SAS) to override contention scheduling and heighten a schema's level of activation to achieve a novel goal.

3. The pre-frontal cortex coordinates executive processing. Recent functional neuro-imaging studies suggest division of the pre-frontal cortex for separable sub-processes. The lateral pre-frontal cortex is a working memory system which selects task relevant information for realistic goal setting. The anterior cingulate cortex sustains attention and monitors competition between cognitive resources in task performance. The medial frontal cortex interacts with the limbic system in the emotional evaluation of behaviour and social decision making.

4. Dysexecutive syndrome (DES) presents as a variety of symptoms, including the inability to plan and organise behaviour. DES is seen after damage to the pre-frontal cortex, often as a result of traumatic brain injury. Inability to reach goals may stem from the loss of processing by the supervisory attention system. Performance skills are affected by poor adaptation, stimulus bound rigidity and perseveration. Inappropriate social behaviour affects relationships with family and carers, and leads to poor prospects for employment.

References

Almeida, Q.J., Black, S. & Roy, E.A. (2002) Screening for apraxia: a short assessment for stroke patients. *Brain and Cognition*, **48**, 253–258.

American Occupational Therapy Association (2002) Occupational Therapy Practice Framework: domain and process. *American Journal of Occupational Therapy*, **56** (6), 609–639.

Andrewes, D. (2001) Disorders of perception. Chapter 2. In: *Neuropsychology: From Theory to Practice*. Psychology Press, Hove.

Assessment of Motor and Process Skills (1998) AMPS Training Manual, Wiltshire: AMPS, UK.

Ayres, A.J. (1985) *Developmental Dyspraxia and Adult-onset Apraxia*. A lecture prepared for Sensory Integration International, Torrance, Calif.

Baddeley, A. (2000) The episodic buffer: a new component of working memory? *Trends in Cognitive Sciences*, **4** (11), 417–423.

Baddeley, A.D. & Hitch, G. (1974) Working memory. In: *The Psychology of Learning and Motivation* (ed. G.H. Bower), Vol. 8, pp. 48–79. Academic Press, London.

Baddeley, A.D., Kopelman, M.D. & Wilson, B.A. (eds) (2002) *Handbook of Memory Disorders*. John Wiley, New York.

Bell, A.R. & Murray, B.J. (2004) Improvement in upper limb performance following stroke: the use of mental practice. *British Journal of Occupational Therapy*, **67** (11) 501–506.

Bilbao, A., Kennedy, C., Chatterji, S., Ustun, B., Barquero, J.L. & Barth, J.T. (2003) The ICF: applications of the WHO model of functioning, disability and health to brain injury rehabilitation. *NeuroRehabilitation*, **18** (3), 239–250.

Bisiach, E. & Luzatti, C. (1978) Unilateral neglect of representational space. *Cortex*, **14**, 129–133.

Borst, M.J. & Peterson, C.Q. (1993) Overcoming topographical orientation deficits in an elderly woman with right cerebrovascular accident. *American Journal of Occupational Therapy*, **47** (6), 551–554.

Bruce, V. & Young, A.W. (1986) Understanding face recognition. *Journal of Psychology*, **77**, 305–327.

Burgess, P.W. & Shallice, T. (1996) Response suppression, initiation and strategy use following frontal lobe lesions. *Neuropsychologica*, **34**, 263–273.

Butler, J. (2002) How comparable are tests of apraxia? *Clinical Rehabilitation*, **16** (4), 389–398.

Cate, Y. & Richards, L. (2000) Relationship between performance on tests of basic visual functions and visual-perceptual processing in persons after brain injury. *American Journal of Occupational Therapy*, **54**, 326–334.

Chen, C.C. (1995) A literature review of constructional performance in adults and children. *Occupational Therapy and Health Care*, **9** (2/3), 145–158.

Christianson, C.H. & Baum, C.M. (eds) (1997) *Occupational Therapy: Enabling Function and Well-being*. Slack, Thorofare, New Jersey.

Cicerone, K.D., Dahlberg, C., Kalmar, K. *et al.* (2000) Evidence-based cognitive rehabilitation: recommendations for clinical practice. *Archives of Physical Medicine and Rehabilitation*, **81** (12, Dec.), 1596–1615.

Cicerone, K., Levin, H., Malec, J., Stuss, D. & Whyte, J. (2006) Cognitive rehabilitation interventions for executive function: moving from bench to bedside in patients with traumatic brain injury. *Journal of Cognitive Neuroscience*, **18** (7, July), 1212–1222.

Clive-Lowe, de, S. (1996) Outcome measurement, cost-effectiveness and clinical audit: the importance of standardised assessment to occupational therapists in meeting these new demands. *British Journal of Occupational Therapy*, **59** (8, Aug.), 357–362.

Cohen, G., Kiss, G. & LeVoi, M. (1993) *Memory: Current Issues*. Open University Press, Buckingham.

College of Occupational Therapists (2004) *Guidance for the Use of the International Classification of Functioning, Disability and Health (ICF) and the Ottawa Charter for Health Promotion in Occupational Therapy Services*. College of Occupational Therapists, London.

College of Occupational Therapists (2005) *Code of Ethics and Professional Conduct*. College of Occupational Therapists, London.

Concha, M.E. (1987) A review of apraxia. *British Journal of Occupational Therapy*, **50** (7), 222–226.

Corbett, A. & Shah, S. (1996) Body scheme disorders following stroke. *British Journal of Occupational Therapy*, **59**, 325–329.

Corbetta, M. & Shulman, G.L. (2002) Control of goal-directed and stimulus-driven attention in the brain. *Nature Reviews Neuroscience*, **3**, 201–215.

Craik, F.I.M. & Tulving, E. (1975) Depth of processing and the retention of words in episodic memory. *Journal of Experimental Psychology, General,* **104**, 268–294.

Crepeau, E.B., Cohn, E.S. & Schell, B.B. (eds) (2003) *Willard and Spackman's Occupational Therapy,* tenth edition. Lippincott, Williams & Wilkins, Philadelphia.

Dahl, T. (2001) *ICF as Framework to Improve Patient Discharge Information – a Study of Patients with Severe Head Injuries Discharged from Intensive Rehabilitation Care.* WHO/GPE/CAS/C/01.47. World Health Organisation, Bethesda, Md.

Damasio, A.R. (1994) *Descartes' Error: Emotion, Reason and the Human Brain.* G.P. Putman, New York.

Desimone, R. & Duncan, J. (1995) Neural mechanisms of selective visual attention. *Annual Review of Neuroscience,* **18**, 193–222.

Donkervoort, M., Dekker, J., Stehmann-Saris, F. & Deelman, B. (2001) Efficacy of strategy training in left hemisphere stroke patients with apraxia: a randomised control trial. *Neuropsychological Rehabilitation,* **11** (5), 549–566.

Donnelly, S.M., Hextell, D.L. & Matthey, S. (1998) The Rivermead Perceptual Assessment Battery: its relationship to selected functional activities. *British Journal of Occupational Therapy,* **61**, 27–32.

Duncan, J. (1986) Disorganisation of behaviour after frontal lobe damage. *Cognitive Neuropsychology,* **3** (3), 271–290.

Edmans, J.A. & Lincoln, N.B. (1990) The relation between perceptual deficits after stroke and independence in activities of daily living. *British Journal of Occupational Therapy,* **53**, 139–142.

Edmans, J., Champion, A., Hill, L. *et al.* (2001) *Occupational Therapy and Stroke.* Stroke Clinical Forum, National Association of Neurological Occupational Therapists. Whurr Publishers, London and Philadelphia.

Ellis, A.W. & Young, A.W. (1988) *Human Cognitive Neuropsychology.* Lawrence Erlbaum, London.

Eslinger, P.J. & Damasio, A.R. (1985) Severe disturbance of higher cognition following bilateral frontal lobe ablation. *Neurology,* **35**, 1731–1741.

Evans, J.J., Wilson, B.A., Schuri, U. *et al.* (2000) A comparison of 'errorless' and 'trial-and-error' learning methods for teaching individuals with acquired memory deficits. *Neuropsychological Rehabilitation,* **10** (1, January), 67–101.

Farah, M.J. (1991) Patterns of co-occurrence among associative agnosias: implications for visual object representation. *Cognitive Neuropsychology,* **8**, 1–19.

Fisher, A.G. (1997) *Assessment of Motor Process Skills,* second edition. Three Star, Fort Collins, Colo.

Fleming, J.M., Shum, D., Strong, J. & Lightbody, S. (2005) Prospective memory rehabilitation for adults with traumatic brain injury: a compensatory training programme. *Brain Injury*, **19** (1), 1–10.

Flinn, N.A. & Radomski, M.V. (2002) Learning. Chapter 12. In: *Occupational Therapy for Physical Dysfunction* (eds C.A. Trombly & M.V. Radomski), fifth edition. Lippincott Williams & Wilkins, Philadelphia.

Gainotti, G., Derme, P., Monteleone, D. & Silveri, M.C. (1986) Mechanisms of unilateral spatial neglect in relation to laterality of cerebral lesions. *Brain*, **109**, 599–612.

Gazzaniga, M.S., Ivry, R.B. & Mangun, G.R. (2002) *Cognitive Neuroscience. The Biology of the Mind.* W.W. Norton & Company, New York.

Geschwind, N. (1975) The apraxias: neural mechanisms of disorders of learned movements. *American Scientist*, **63**, 188–195.

Gibson, J.J. (1979) *The Ecological Approach to Visual Perception.* Houghton Miffin, Boston.

Goldenberg, G. & Hagman, S. (1998) Therapy of activities of daily living in patients with apraxia. *Clinical Rehabilitation*, **8** (2), 123–141.

Goldenberg, G., Daumuller, M. & Hagmann, S. (2001) Assessment and therapy of complex activities of daily living in apraxia. *Neuropsychological Rehabilitation*, **11** (2), 147–169.

Goodale, M.A. & Milner, A.D. (1992) Separate visual pathways for perception and action. *Trends in Neurosciences*, **15**, 20–25.

Groome, D. (1999) *An Introduction to Cognitive Psychology. Processes and Disorders.* Psychology Press, Hove.

Haaland, K.Y., Harrington, D.L. & Knight, R.T. (2000) Neural representations of skilled movement. *Brain*, **123**, 2306–2313.

Haglund, L., Henriksson, C., Crisp, M., Friedheim, L. & Kielhofner, G. (2001) Cited in Introduction to evaluation and interviewing. Chapter 22. In: *Willard and Spackman's Occupational Therapy* (eds E.B. Crepeau, E.B. Cohn & B.B. Schell), tenth edition. Lippincott Williams & Wilkins, Philadelphia.

Halligan, P.W. & Marshall, J.C. (1991) Left neglect for near but not far space in man. *Nature*, **350**, 498–500.

Halligan, P.W. & Marshall, J.C. (1994) Toward a principled explanation of unilateral neglect. *Cognitive Neuropsychology*, **11**, 167–206.

Hanna-Pladdy, B. & Gonzales Rothi, L.J. (2001) Ideational apraxia: confusion that began with Liepman. *Neuropsychological Rehabilitation*, **11** (5), 539–547.

Hanna-Pladdy, B., Heilman, K.M. & Foundas, A.L. (2001) Cortical and sub-cortical contributions to ideomotor apraxia. *Brain*, **124**, 2513–2527.

Hartman-Maeir, A. & Katz, N. (1995) Validity of the Behavioural Inattention Test (BIT): relationships with functional tasks. *American Journal of Occupational Therapy*, **49**, 507–516.

Heilman, K.M. & Valenstein, E. (1993) *Clinical Neuropsychology*. Oxford University Press, New York.

Hobart, J.C., Lamping, D.L. & Thompson, A.J. (1996) Evaluating neurological outcome measures: the bare essentials. Editorial. *Journal of Neurology, Neurosurgery & Psychiatry*, **60**, 127–130.

Hocking, C. (2001) Implementing occupation-based assessment. *American Journal of Occupational Therapy*, **55** (4), 463–469.

Humphreys, G.W. & Riddoch, M.J. (1987) *To See but Not to See. A case study of visual agnosia*. London, Erlbaum.

Jackson, T. (1999) Dyspraxia: guidelines for intervention. *British Journal of Occupational Therapy*, **62** (7), 321–326.

Jonides, J., Smith, E.E., Koeppe, R.A., Awh, E., Minoshima, S. & Mintun, M.A. (1993) Spatial working memory in humans as revealed by PET. *Nature*, **363**, 623–624.

Kahneman, D. (1973) *Attention and Effort*. Prentice-Hall, New Jersey.

Karlsson, G. (1993) *Psychological Qualitative Research from a Phenomenological Perspective*. Almquist & Wiksell, Stockholm.

Katz, N. & Hartman-Maeir, A. (1997) Occupational performance and metacognition. *Canadian Journal of Occupational Therapy*, **64** (2), 53–62.

Lampinen, J. & Tham, K. (2003) Interaction with the physical environment in everyday occupation after stroke: a phenomenological study of persons with visuo-spatial agnosia. *Scandinavian Journal of Occupational Therapy*, **10**, 147–156.

Laver, A.J. & Powell, G. (1995) *The Structured Observational Test of Function*. Nfer-Nelson, Windsor.

Law, M., Polatajko, H., Baptiste, W. & Townsend, E. (1997) Core concepts of occupational therapy. In: *Enabling Occupation: an Occupational Therapy Perspective* (ed. E. Townsend), pp. 29–56. Canadian Association of Occupational Therapists, Ottawa, Ontario.

Law, M., Baptiste, S., Carswell, A., McColl, M.A., Polatajko, H. & Pollock, N. (1998) The Canadian Occupational Performance Measure: an outcome measure for occupational therapy. *Canadian Journal of Occupational Therapy*, **57**, 82–87.

Lee, S.S., Powell, N. & Esdaile, S. (2001) A functional model of cognitive rehabilitation in occupational therapy. *Canadian Journal of Occupational Therapy*, **68** (1), 41–50.

Levy, L.L. (2001) Memory processing and the older adult: what practitioners need to know. *Occupational Therapy Practice*, **6** (7), 1–8.

Lin, K. (1996) Right hemispheric activation approaches to neglect rehabilitation post-stroke. *American Journal of Occupational Therapy*, **50**, 504–515.

Lincoln, N.B., Majid, M.J. & Weyman, N. (2000) Cognitive rehabilitation for attention deficits following stroke. *Cochrane Database of Systematic Reviews*, Issue 4. Art. No. CD002842. DOI: 10.1002/14651858.CD002842.

Luria, A.R. (1966) *The Higher Cortical Functions in Man*. Basic Books, New York.

McColl, M.A., Law, M., Stewart, D., Doubt, L., Pollock, N. & Krupa, T. (2003) *Theoretical Basis of Occupational Therapy*, second edition. Slack Inc., Thorafare, New Jersey.

Maddicks, R., Marzillier, S.L. & Parker, G. (2003) Rehabilitation of unilateral neglect in the acute recovery stage: the efficacy of limb activation therapy. *Neuropsychological Rehabilitation*, **13** (3), 391–408.

Maguire, E.A., Frackowiak, R.S.J. & Frith, C.D. (1997) Recalling routes around London: activation of the right hippocampus in taxi drivers. *Journal of Neuroscience*, **17**, 7103–7110.

Maguire, E.A., Burgess, N., Donnett, J.G., Frackowiak, R.S.J., Frith, C.D. & O' Keefe, J. (1998) Knowing where and getting there: a human navigation network. *Science*, **280**, 921–924.

Marr, D. (1982) *Vision: a Computational Investigation into the Human Representation and Processing of Visual Information*. Freeman, San Francisco.

Miller, N. (1986) *Dyspraxia and its Management*. Croom Helm, London.

Milner, B. (1963) Effects of different brain lesions on card sorting. *Archives of Neurology*, **9**, 90–100.

Niemeier, J., Kreutzer, J. & Taylor, L. (2005) Acute cognitive and neurobehavioural intervention for individuals with acquired brain injury: preliminary outcome data. *Neuropsychological Rehabilitation*, **15** (2, May), 129–146.

Norman, D.A. (1980) Twelve issues for cognitive science. *Cognitive Science*, **4**, 1–32.

Norris, G. & Tate, R.L. (2000) The Behavioural Assessment of the Dysexecutive Syndrome (BADS): ecological, concurrent and construct validity. *Neuropsychological Rehabilitation*, **10** (1, January), 33–45.

Paulescu, E., Frith, C.D. & Frackowiak, R.S.J. (1993) The neural correlates of the verbal component of working memory. *Nature*, **362**, 342–345.

Posner, M.I. & Peterson, S.E. (1990) The attention system of the human brain. *Annual Review of Neuroscience*, **13**, 25–42.

Quintana, L.A. (2002) Vision and visual perception. Chapter 7. In: *Occupational Therapy for Physical Dysfunction* (eds C.A. Trombley & M.V. Radomski), fifth edition. Lippincott, Williams and Wilkins, Philadelphia.

Radomski, M.V. (2002) Chapter 8. In: *Occupational Therapy for Physical Dysfunction* (eds C.A. Trombley & M.V. Radomski), fifth edition. Lippincott, Williams and Wilkins, Philadelphia.

Riddoch M.J. & Humphreys G.W. (1987) Visual object processing in a case of semantic access agnosia. *Cognitive Neuropsychology*, **4**, 131–185.

Robertson, I.H. & North, N. (1992) Active and passive activation of left limbs: influence on visual and sensory neglect. *Neuropsychologica*, **31**, 293–300.

Robertson, I.H., Hogg, K. & McMillan, T.M. (1998) Rehabilitation of unilateral neglect: improving function by contralesional limb activation. *Neuropsychological Rehabilitation*, **8**, 19–29.

Robertson, L.C. & Lamb, M.R. (1991) Neuropsychological contributions to theories of part/whole organisation. *Cognitive Psychology*, **23**, 299–330.

Roy, E.A. (1996) Hand preference, manual asymmetries and limb apraxia. Chapter 11. In: *Manual Asymmetries in Motor Performance* (eds D. Elliott & E.A. Roy). CRC Press, Boston.

Roy, E.A. & Square, P.A. (1994) Neuropsychology of movement sequencing disorders and apraxia. In: *Neuropsychology* (ed. D.W. Zaidel), pp. 185–214. Academic Press, San Diego.

Sacks, O. (1985) *The Man who Mistook his Wife for a Hat*. Duckworth, London.

Salter, K., Jutai, J.W., Teasell, R., Foley, N.C. & Bitensky, J. (2005a) Issues for selection of outcome measures in stroke rehabilitation: ICF body functions. *Disability and Rehabilitation*, **27** (4), 191–207.

Salter, K., Jutai, J.W., Teasell, R., Foley, N.C., Bitensky, J. & Bayley, M. (2005b) Issues for selection of outcome measures in stroke rehabilitation: ICF activity. *Disability and Rehabilitation*, **27** (6), 315–340.

Salter, K., Jutai, J.W., Teasell, R., Foley, N.C., Bitensky, J. & Bayley, M. (2005c) Issues for selection of outcome measures in stroke rehabilitation: ICF participation. *Disability and Rehabilitation*, **27** (9), 507–528.

Saver, J.L. & Damasio, A.R. (1991) Preserved access and processing of social knowledge in a patient with acquired sociopathology due to frontal damage. *Neuropsychologica*, **29**, 1241–1249.

Shallice, T. (1982) Specific impairment of planning. *Philosophical Transactions of the Royal Society of London B*, **298**, 199–209.

Shallice, T. & Burgess, P.W. (1991) Deficits in strategy application following frontal lobe damage in man. *Brain*, **114**, 727–741.

Sirigu, A., Grafman, J., Bressler, K. & Sunderland, T. (1991) Multiple representations contribute to body knowledge processing: evidence from a case of autopagnosia. *Brain*, **114**, 629–642.

Sohlberg, M.M., Mateer, C. & Stuss, D.T. (1993) Contemporary approaches to the management of executive control dysfunction. *Journal of Head Trauma Rehabilitation*, **8** (1), 45–58.

Spelke, E.S., Hirst, W.C. & Neisser, U. (1976) Skills of divided attention. *Cognition*, **4**, 215–230.

Stirling, J. (2002) *Introducing Neuropsychology*. Psychology Press, Hove.

Styles, E.A. (1997) *The Psychology of Attention*. Psychology Press, Hove.

Tate, R.L. & McDonald S. (1995) What is apraxia? The clinician's dilemma. *Neuropsychological Rehabilitation*, **5** (4), 273–297.

Tham, K., Borell, L. & Gustavsson, A. (2000) The discovery of disability: a phenomenological study of unilateral neglect. *American Journal of Occupational Therapy*, **54**, 398–406.

Titus, M.N.D., Gall, N.G., Yerxa, E.J., Roberson, T.A. & Mack, W. (1991) Correlation of perceptual performance and activities of daily living in stroke patients. *American Journal of Occupational Therapy*, **45**, 410–418.

Toglia, J.P. (1989) Visual perception of objects. An approach to assessment and intervention. *American Journal of Occupational Therapy*, **43**, 587–595.

Toglia, J.P. (1991) Generalisation of Treatment: A Multi Context Approach to Cognitive Perceptual Impairment in Adults with Brain Injury. *American Journal of Occupational Therapy*, **45** (6), 505–516.

Treisman, A. & Gelade, G. (1980) A feature integration theory of attention. *Cognitive Psychology*, **12**, 97–136.

Trombley, C.A. & Radomski, M.V. (eds) (2002) *Occupational Therapy for Physical Dysfunction*, fifth edition. Lippincott Williams & Wilkins, Baltimore, Md.

Tulving, E. (1997) Organisation of memory: *quo vadis?* In: *Conversations in Cognitive Neuroscience* (ed. M.S. Gazzaniga), No. 54. MIT Press, Cambridge, Mass.

Wade, D.T. (2004) Assessment, measurement and data collection tools. Editorial. *Clinical Rehabilitation*, **18**, 233–237.

Walker, C.M. & Walker, M.F. (2001) Dressing ability after stroke: a review of the literature. *British Journal of Occupational Therapy*, **64** (9), 449–454.

Whiting, S., Lincoln, N.B., Bhavnani, G. & Cockburn, J. (1985) *The Rivermead Perceptual Assessment Battery*. NFER-Nelson, Windsor.

Wilson, B.A. & Wearing, D. (1995) Amnesia in a musician. In: *Broken Memories: Case Studies in Memory Impairment* (eds R. Campbell & M. Conway). Blackwell, Oxford.

Wilson, F.C. & Manly, T. (2003) Sustained attention training and errorless learning facilitates self-care functioning in chronic ipsilesional neglect following severe traumatic brain injury. *Neuropsychological Rehabilitation*, **13** (5, December), 537–548.

World Health Organisation (1946) Constitution of the World Health Organisation. *American Journal Public Health Nations Health*, **36** (11, November), 1315–1323.

World Health Organisation (2001) *International Classification of Functioning, Disability and Health*. World Health Organisation, Geneva.

Ylvisaker, M. & Szekeres, S.F. (1989) Metacognitive and executive impairments in head-injured children and adults. *Topics in Language Disorders*, **9** (2), 34–49.

York, C.D. & Cermak, S.A. (1995) Visual perception and praxis in adults after stroke. *American Journal of Occupational Therapy*, **49** (6), 543–550.

Young, A.W., Hay, D.C. & Ellis, A.W. (1985) The faces that launched a thousand slips: everyday difficulties and errors in recognising people. *British Journal of Psychology*, **76**, 495– 523.

Zihl, J., Von Cramon, D. & Mai, N. (1983) Selective disturbance of movement vision after bilateral brain damage. *Brain*, **106**, 313–340.

Zoccolatti, P. & Judica, A. (1991) Functional evaluation of hemineglect by means of a semi-structured scale. *Neuropsychological Rehabilitation*, **1**, 33–44.

Zoltan, B. (1996) *Vision, Perception and Cognition: a Manual for the Evaluation and Treatment of the Neurologically Impaired Adult*. Slack Inc., Thorofare, New Jersey.

Zwinkels, A., Geusgens, C., Van de Sande, P. & Van Heugten, C. (2004) Assessment of apraxia: inter-rater reliability of a new apraxia test, association between apraxia and other cognitive deficits and prevalence of apraxia in a rehabilitation setting. *Clinical Rehabilitation*, **18**, 819–827.

Glossary

The prefixes 'a' and 'dys' are used interchangeably in describing deficits. Their literal meanings are 'inability to' and 'impairment of', respectively.

achromatopsia   inability to recognise colour, in the absence of retinal defects.

activity   the execution of a task or action by an individual (ICF). Occupational therapists commonly define activity as the purposeful execution of one or more related tasks leading to the achievement of a goal. Activities, related in time, context or purpose, form areas of occupation, for example self-care, work, or leisure (OTPF).

activity demands (OTPF)   the elements required for the successful execution of an activity including the spatial, temporal, social and cultural aspects, and the body structures, body functions and performance skills.

activity limitations (ICF)   difficulties an individual may have in executing activities, resulting from impairments, or from environmental barriers and constraints.

affordance   possibility for action provided by a surface or an object.

agnosia   inability to recognise familiar objects, in the absence of sensory impairment.

   apperceptive   failure to recognise familiar objects as a result of visual perceptual impairment.

   associative (semantic)   inability to integrate object percept with knowledge of object meaning and function.

agraphia   inability to produce meaningful written words.

alexia   reading disorder.

allocentric   spatial representations of the environment, irrespective of body position.

amnesia   partial or complete loss of memory.

   amnesic syndrome   global deterioration in memory function due to non-degenerative brain lesion.

anterograde   difficulty in remembering new information acquired after brain damage.

retrograde   loss of memory for a variable period of time prior to the onset of brain damage.

anomia   inability to name objects and faces.

anosognosia   inability to recognise a part of one's own body.

aphasia   inability to process spoken language.

apraxia (dyspraxia)   inability to make purposeful movements (in the presence of normal sensation and muscle tone).

ideational   loss of the concept of movement (i.e. semantic knowledge related to action).

ideomotor   disorder in the timing and spatial organisation of purposeful movement.

arousal   physiological level of attention based on the activity in the reticular formation of the brain stem.

articulatory loop   subvocal rehearsal of speech-based information in working memory.

assessment   the process of establishing the health status and function of an individual or group. Assessment involves the selection and use of a range of methods and tools at the commencement of intervention to establish strengths, difficulties and needs. This informs intervention planning. Reassessment may be carried out during and at completion of intervention, as a part of outcome measurement.

astereognosis (tactile agnosia)   inability to recognise objects from touch without vision.

attention   active processing directed to particular sensory stimuli for perceptual and semantic analysis.

divided   ability to divide attention between two or more activities that are competing.

selective   processing in which a person selectively attends to certain high priority environmental stimuli in preference to others.

sustained (vigilance)   attention maintained over prolonged periods of time or in repetitive activity.

autobiographical memory   long-term memory that is unique to the individual.

Balint syndrome   a condition in which some people with brain damage find it difficult to shift visual attention.

ballistic movement (see **open loop**)   action that is pre-programmed and cannot be modified once it has begun.

barriers (to performance) (ICF)   contexts or contextual factors that create difficulties for people, or prevent performance of tasks, activities and occupations. Negative attitudes or stigmas associated with disability are barriers that may prevent engagement in life situations and occupations. Physical barriers such as stairs and high-set lift buttons prevent wheelchair access and movement around a building.

biopsychosocial   an adjective used to describe a frame of reference in which biological, psychological and social theories of human function are all considered relevant to health and occupational performance. Working within a frame of reference leads to the selection of models and frameworks of practice compatible with it.

body functions (ICF)   all the physiological functions of the body and its component structures. These include psychological functions. Body functions are classified as 'client factors' by the OTPF.

body image   subjective perception of the appearance of one's own body.

body scheme   perception of the relative position of the body parts.

body structures (ICF)   anatomical parts of the body such as limbs, organs and tissues. Body structures are classified as 'client factors' by the OTPF.

bottom-up assessment   the focus on the impairment of components of the cognitive system which affect occupational performance.

bottom-up processing   is directly influenced by environmental stimuli before further processing.

capacity (ICF)   is highest probable level at which an individual is able to perform a given task or activity. Capacity is best determined in an environment which is free of factors that might impact upon performance, or in which such factors are controllable or measurable. Cognitive function depends on the allocation of resources from the information processing capacity of the brain. The total capacity is reduced in people with brain damage.

CAT scan   computerised axial tomography. A thin fan-shaped X-ray beam views a 'slice' of the brain. The X-ray tube revolves round the patient so that the brain is viewed from all angles. A computer combines all the views, and the changes in soft tissue at the lesion site are revealed in a single image.

central executive   control system that allocates attention between the visuo-spatial and phonological components of working memory.

cerebrovascular accident (event) (CVA) a rapidly developing focal lesion in the brain that is vascular in origin.

closed loop action that is modified during progress in response to internal and external feedback.

'cocktail party phenomenon' the way we attend to some stimuli and ignore others.

coding mental processing of information during learning.

cognitive system a set of mental operations performed to reach a common goal.

colour constancy tendency for a colour to look the same under a wide variation of lighting and viewing conditions.

concept the stored mental representations of a set of objects, actions or events that share certain characteristics.

confabulation the report of memories which the person believes to be true but they are false.

constructional apraxia difficulty in the organisation of complex actions in two- or three-dimensional space.

contention scheduling mechanism for the activation of a stored schema, triggered by the environment, with inhibition of competing schemas.

context the particular circumstances in which an event or action takes place.

contextual factors (OTPF,ICF) all the factors which make up the total environment in which people live and conduct their lives, and which impact upon the ability to carry out tasks, activities, roles and occupations. Contexts include the physical, social and attitudinal environment, and personal factors such as gender, age and education.

declarative memory long-term memory for facts, incidents and events that are retrieved by conscious access.

dissociation the separation of one module of processing that is impaired when others are spared.

double dissociation two modules of processing which can be selectively impaired.

dressing apraxia inability to dress oneself, primarily due to a disorder of spatial perception and/or body scheme.

dysexecutive syndrome impairment of the executive functions of the brain which is associated with frontal lobe lesion.

episodic memory long-term memories linked to a time and place.

executive functions   the mental operations involved in: goal-setting, organising, monitoring and completing, action and behaviour.

central executive   a component of working memory.

explicit memory   memory processes with awareness, assessed by tests of direct recall and recognition.

facilitators (of performance) (ICF)   contexts or contextual factors that support and enable performance of a task, activity or occupation. Physical environmental factors such as ramps facilitate access for wheelchair users. Anti-discrimination legislation facilitates employment of people with disabilities.

figure ground   the isolation of a shape or an object from its background.

form constancy   the perception of a familiar shape or object as the same, regardless of its position or the distance from which it is viewed.

framework (of practice)   sometimes used interchangeably with 'model'. A framework refers to the definition and organisation of a set of related ideas and concepts drawn from specific theories. A framework can be used to structure and analyse information, provide a common lexicon, determine priorities for intervention and guide problem solving (ICF, OTPF).

gestalt   unified whole that is not revealed by simply analysing the parts.

gesture   a meaningful action. Gestures are divided into types for the assessment of praxis.

imitation   a gesture made by an examiner is copied by a subject either at the same time or after an interval.

pantomime   a mime of a gesture is performed by a subject on command.

transitive   using an object held in the hand.

intransitive   does not involve an object, for example wave goodbye.

hemianopia   'blindness' in part of the visual field of one or both eyes, originating in the pathway from the retina to the occipital cortex.

homonymous hemianopia   'blindness' in the right or left side visual fields of both eyes.

hemiplegia   weakness or spasticity in the muscles of one side of the body, resulting from a lesion in the opposite side of the brain.

hippocampus   a buried gyrus in the temporal lobe of the brain involved in memory and spatial orientation.

impairments   problems of body structure or function such as abnormality, deviation, or loss (ICF). Impairments of cognitive function originate in the loss of information processing at any level, or in the access to that level, in the cognitive system.

implicit memory   memory that is not directly revealed in tests of recall and recognition.

lesion (brain)   change in the tissue of the brain resulting from vascular accident, trauma, disease or degeneration.

lexicon   store of known words.

long-term memory   memory that stores and processes information over periods of time from a few minutes to many years.

memory trace   neurological processing for a relatively permanent memory.

metacognition   a person's belief and knowledge about his or her own cognitive processes or 'knowing what you know'.

modality   a sensory system, for example visual modality, tactile modality.

model (of practice)   seeks to describe and explain human health and behaviour according to one or more theories. It incorporates and defines concepts, and directs the therapist to select particular goals, approaches and methods of intervention.

module   a core stage in information processing which may or may not relate to activity in a specific brain area.

MRI   magnetic resonance imaging. A strong magnetic field is produced by electromagnets distributed around the head. A radio pulse excites the hydrogen atoms in the water in the brain tissue. A computer translates the signals from the movement of the hydrogen atoms into an image, which identifies where lesions have occurred.

myelin   fatty sheath around axons of neurones in the white matter of the central nervous system, and in peripheral nerves, which increases the rate of conduction of nerve impulses.

neglect syndrome   failure to orient, report or respond to stimuli on one side of space (contralateral to the side of brain lesion).

neuro-imaging   scanning techniques which show the structure and/or the rate of local blood flow in brain areas; see CAT, MRI and PET scanning.

object-centred description representation of the visual structure of an object, irrespective of viewpoint.

object constancy the tendency for objects to be perceived as the same, even though they are observed in a variety of conditions, for example distance, orientation, location or lighting.

object-recognition units stored visual descriptions of all known objects.

occupational form refers to the set of observable components and features that comprise an occupation; what the person actually does when carrying out an occupation (rather than what meaning it has or what function it is serving).

open loop movement that cannot be modified once it has started, for example tap a key on a computer keyboard, throw a ball.

optic aphasia inability to name objects when presented visually, but can name from a verbal description and can gesture the use of the object.

optic ataxia inability to use the visual information from objects to guide action in the presence of intact object recognition.

outcome the degree of change that has occurred to specified characteristics of a person, population or situation as a consequence of therapeutic intervention.

outcome measures tools used to determine and measure the change that has occurred in a person, population or situation, as a result of intervention. Some outcome measures are used as assessment tools throughout the intervention process as well as at the end, to provide a measure of change over time.

paradigm a particular experimental procedure that is described in detail.

parallel processing when two or more cognitive processes occur at the same time.

participation (ICF) involvement in life situations. May be equated with 'roles' (OTPF) in which individuals engage in a set of behaviours having socially agreed and recognised functions, for example parent, worker, church elder.

participation restrictions (ICF) problems and difficulties an individual may experience in involvement in life situations, or in the execution of roles and occupations.

performance (ICF) what a person actually does when carrying out a task or activity within the usual or current context.

performance objectives statements of desired outcomes of occupational interventions. Objectives are descriptions of observable behaviours that are specific, measurable, achievable and timely, such that their attainment or non-attainment provides a measure of progress towards a goal.

performance patterns (OTPF)   patterns of behaviour related to daily life activities and occupations.

habits   automatic behaviours that support performance of tasks and activities.

routines   sets of activities that occur in an established sequence and support execution of roles and occupations.

roles   sets of behaviours that have socially agreed and recognised functions.

performance skills (OTPF)   component elements of what an individual does, related to functional purposes. The coordinated action of body functions in the performance of tasks and activities.

perseveration   tendency to continue a particular action, word or pattern of behaviour, when the stimulus has been removed.

phonological store   temporary storage of speech-based information in working memory.

positron emission tomography, PET scan   reveals the level of activity in the different areas of the brain over time. A solution containing a radioactive isotope is injected intravenously and accumulates in the brain in amounts proportional to the local blood flow. The positrons emitted by the isotope are detected by sensors placed around the head.

praxis   means, literally, movement. In neuropsychology the term applies to meaningful actions and gestures.

pre-frontal cortex   area of the frontal lobe anterior to the motor areas, associated with the executive functions.

procedural memory   long-term memory for mental and motor skills that are retrieved without conscious awareness.

prosopagnosia   inability to recognise familiar faces, in the presence of intact visual perception and object recognition.

prospective memory   memory for future actions without obvious external cues.

representation   neural activity in the processing of a member of a conceptual category.

stored memory   as it has been in the past.

structural   as it is now.

saccade   a fast eye movement between two fixation points, occurring in scanning and reading.

scanning   the exploration of space by eye movements.

schema   organised packets of information about places, events or people stored in long-term memory.

semantic   related to meaning.

semantic memory   long-term memory for general knowledge and facts.

serial processing   when one process is completed before the next one starts.

somatognosia   failure to perceive how the body parts relate to each other, and their relative positions in space (disorder of body scheme).

standardized assessment tool   a published measurement tool designed for use with a specific population and for a specified purpose. Instructions are provided to ensure consistency of administration, scoring and interpretation of results. Evidence of validity and reliability is available through published studies.

structural description   specification of the parts of an object and the way they fit together; a framework for object recognition.

sulcus   a fold in the surface of the brain.
   central   separates the frontal and parietal lobes.
   lateral   separates the temporal lobe from the frontal and parietal lobes

supervisory attention system   system for controlled attention in novel situations, or when decision making is required.

syndrome   a collection of symptoms that commonly occur together.

therapeutic approach   the utilisation of a range of intervention methods and techniques that have a common theoretical basis. The therapeutic approach may also determine the choice of assessment and outcome measures.

top-down assessment   the focus on occupational roles and performance as a basis for compensation and adaptation in occupational therapy intervention.

top-down processing   sequence of processes for the interpretation of information from the senses that are influenced by stored knowledge from past experience.

topographical disorientation   inability to recall the spatial arrangement of familiar surroundings.

topographical memory   memory for the landmarks and layout of familiar surroundings.

transcranial magnetic stimulation TMS   technique used to explore the effects of brief stimulation of the cortical areas of the brain. An electric current is applied in a coil placed on the skin over the brain area of interest.

unilateral visual neglect   inability to orient to visual stimuli in one side of space.

utilisation behaviour   tendency to pick up and use objects in close proximity that are clearly not appropriate to the task in hand.

viewer-centred representation   visual representation of an object from the viewpoint of the observer.

visual field   area of the visual world that is visible out of the eye.

visuo-spatial sketchpad   processing of visuo-spatial information in working memory.

working memory   temporary storage of visuo-spatial and speech-based information controlled by an attentional system (central executive).

Index